To Antony

Best Wishes

from

Mavis

RELEASING THE POWER TO HEAL

A Celebration of 10 Years of Holistic Healing

Mavis Cunningham MA B Ed

Founder of The Cancer Support Centre – Sutton Coldfield

Forward by Professor Jane Plant CBE
Author of *Your Life in Your Hands*

Preface by David Hamilton PhD
Author of *How Your Mind Can Heal Your Body*

All profits from this book will go to
The Cancer Support Centre – Sutton Coldfield

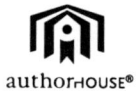

authorHOUSE®

AuthorHouse™ UK Ltd.
500 Avebury Boulevard
Central Milton Keynes, MK9 2BE
www.authorhouse.co.uk
Phone: 08001974150

First published by AuthorHouse 1/10/2011

ISBN: 978-1-4567-7205-5 (sc)

Contents

List of Contribuors

Mavis Cunningham	Founder, Author, Editor & Therapist
Sue Arnold	Yoga Teacher
Anita Bridges	Hypnotherapist, Louise Hay Trainer
Loretto Cattell	Quantum Touch Practitioner, 'M' Technique Trainer
Irene Dorrett	Founder Member & Aromatherapist
Anne Findlay	Walking Group & Book Club Leader
Sheila Greenough	Reiki Master, 'M' Technique Practitioner
Eleanor Hamlett	Founder Member & Aromatherapist
Gill Howell	Art Teacher & Reiki Master
Loraine Hyden	Reflexologist, Reiki Practitioner
Marie Jones	Meditation Group Leader
Louise Kesterton	Acupuncturist
Sue LeBlanc	Hypnotherapist, EFT Practitioner
Toni Lester	Reiki Master/Teacher
Roy Poller	Hypnotherapist
Angela Richmond	Nutritional Advisor
Linda Sutton	Counsellor/Course Leader/Group Facilitator
Sharon Taylor	Indian Head Massage Practitioner
Mike Watson	Bowen Technique Practitioner

Acknowledgements

I would like to thank all my friends and colleagues at The Cancer Support Centre who have encouraged and supported me during the writing of this book, especially those who have contributed to the book by writing about their own therapeutic methods.

I would also like to thank those Cancer Centre clients who have generously allowed me to tell their amazing stories.

My sincere thanks also go to my friend and mentor Easton who has constantly offered his support, encouragement and wisdom.

Foreword

I am very pleased to be writing a foreword to this inspiring book, written to celebrate the tenth anniversary of The Cancer Support Centre- Sutton Coldfield, of which I am proud to be a patron.

I have visited the Centre and experienced the caring atmosphere there and the professional approach to holistic healing. I have talked with some of the complementary therapists and group leaders and become aware of their considerable knowledge, experience and expertise.

This book comprehensively covers the full range of therapies and group activities offered at the Centre. It demonstrates, through the remarkable personal stories, which are included, how the provision of therapeutic services and a caring environment can help people come to terms with and overcome their cancer.

I am delighted that the book includes a detailed chapter on nutrition which endorses my work on the effects dairy products in the promotion of certain cancers and how adopting a dairy free diet can help in the primary prevention or recurrence of cancer.

Professor Jane Plant CBE DSc FRSM
Author of *Your Life in Your Hands* and *The Plant Programme*

Preface

I discovered the Cancer Support Centre in Sutton Coldfield about a year ago when I was invited to give a talk to clients, volunteers and their friends and families. I have been back several times since and have learned more about the wonderful work done there.

The ethos and philosophy of the Centre concurs with many of my own beliefs: the value of positive thinking, relaxation, visualisation and kindness, all of which I have written about in my books, are part of the message and teaching at the Centre. There is a strong belief amongst the therapists that I have met, that 'the mind can heal the body'.

This book with its description of the therapeutic methods offered at the Centre and its remarkable stories of clients' recovery from cancer will be an inspiration to readers to practice positive thinking, relaxation, visualisation and kindness for the benefits of their own healing, health and wellbeing, and also for the prevention of disease.

David Hamilton PhD
Author of *Your Mind Can Heal Your Body* and *Why Kindness Is Good For You*

The History of The Cancer Support Centre

In the latter part of the 1990's, a number of people in Sutton Coldfield were all facing up to their own experiences of cancer. Some were actually living with and learning to cope with the effects of cancer, others were working in a professional capacity with people suffering from cancer, whilst others were caring for family or friends facing the diagnosis of and treatment for various types of cancer. People in these situations were known to me.

I had recently retired from my position as a Lecturer in Nursing and started a new career in counselling and hypnotherapy, so had encountered a number of people affected by cancer. I had also experienced the effects cancer in members of my own family. I was very aware of the effects the diagnosis of cancer had on those being treated for the disease as well as their family members and friends.

Initially in 1998, I talked to a few colleagues, who were counsellors and able to teach relaxation techniques to their clients, and asked them to join me in forming an evening Support and Relaxation Group for all those affected by cancer. This group, which included family members and friends of those with cancer, met fortnightly to share their experiences, enjoy a cup of tea together and learn to relax and use creative visualisation. At the beginning, the group was allowed to meet in the oncology department at the local hospital and we were very grateful to be offered that venue. As time moved on, the group members expressed the wish to meet in a less clinical environment, where they would not be reminded of their experiences in the hospital. The next meeting place was a room in a church centre and this was followed by the offer to use a room at the local Fire Station. This latter venue proved both interesting and a challenge for the group leader as it was not unknown for the fire bell to go off in the middle of a session.

In 2000, recognising the need to develop the Support Group further and recognising the imperfections of the environments being used, I decided to

1

contact by letter all the people I thought would be interested in setting up a Cancer Support Centre in Sutton Coldfield. Some of these had experienced the activities at the, then, Bristol Cancer Help Centre, (now Penny Brohn Centre), but it was a long distance to travel and the costs were too great for many people. Those, who responded to my letter, met to decide on a way forward and became the founder members of the Cancer Support Centre, Sutton Coldfield.

The founder members of the Centre were all in agreement with the aspiration to have a sanctuary where people with cancer and their families and friends could come. It would be a unique place, warm and welcoming, peaceful and tranquil, somewhere relaxing and safe. It would offer support, refreshment, chat and laughter as well as free complementary therapies, counselling and relaxation classes.

Following the setting up of a committee in October 2000, some people started fundraising activities and others became involved in administration and legal activities, commencing the process of obtaining Company and Charitable Status. Company and Registered Charity status were achieved in 2001/2002.

Initially there were three trustees supported by a committee of eight. Over the years the format has changed so that the managing body now consists of just trustees, currently six, although there have been more at some points. Trustees have changed as their term of office expired or have retired for other reasons. In total there have been eighteen different trustees during the ten years, ten of these have been therapists and five have been affected by cancer; some trustees fell into both the above categories. The remainder were volunteers. Other important voluntary posts are treasurer and company secretary. There have been 3 of the former and also 3 of the latter. Those who have had a fundraising responsibility have also been vital to the development of the organisation and there have been a number of these. Currently one voluntary fundraiser leads others in these activities.

There was so much goodwill and kindness from so many people who offered time and financial help, and the dream of a place of our own came to fruition in October 2001, when the Cancer Support Centre opened in a little rented house in Farthing Lane, in the centre of Sutton Coldfield. Initially the Centre opened for one day a week. The house was rather shabby, but with a great deal of creative input and a lot of enthusiasm, it soon felt like home and became greatly loved by many clients. The Centre was now able to offer some individual complementary therapies and self-help courses to clients. After a while the Centre started to open on 2 days a week.

As the numbers of clients grew steadily and demand for complementary therapies increased, it became clear that larger premises were needed. At this point Sutton Coldfield Municipal Charities were consulted and they stepped in with a marvellous offer to fund the rent of larger premises for the Centre for 3 years. This enabled the Cancer Support Centre to move to the seemingly (then) enormous Station House in Midland Drive. This building was originally a railway station on a line which now only carries freight. It had been converted to offices some years before.

Before moving in some alterations were made to improve the environment and to comply with the Equal Opportunities law for access. The weekend before opening, the trustees and committee members had a working party to add furnishings and create a relaxing environment. What a weekend that was! Volunteers moved furniture, plants and books from Farthing Lane. A donor generously provided the Centre with office furniture and the trustees made a trip to a large Swedish store. This was followed by the swift building of lots of flat-packed furniture. There was a great atmosphere developing in the building.

The Cancer Support Centre has now occupied Station House for over 6 years and the services have developed considerably. However the atmosphere of peace and tranquillity, which is often mixed with fun and laughter, still pervades the building.

The Centre is currently open regularly from Monday to Thursday with a programme of individual therapies and group activities every day. The Centre is often open at weekends for training events and courses and in the evening for trustee, therapist and volunteer meetings. The Centre has been staffed since 2005 with a part-time administrator and since 2007 with a part-time Volunteer Coordinator. All other officers and workers are volunteers, who are able to claim appropriate expenses. The building now has inadequate space and insufficient rooms and staff for the services to develop further and the dream is now for a larger building and more staff in the near future.

Fund-raising activities are immensely important to ensure the continuation of the Centre. Numerous applications need to be made to obtain grants from funding bodies and many fund-raising events are planned annually by the fundraiser and her team. The Centre does receive much support from local businesses and sports clubs. All those who support the Centre are invited to visit the centre and see the services in action.

Margaret's Story

Margaret was referred to the Cancer Support Centre in 2004 by her Macmillan Nurse. She had been diagnosed with terminal ovarian cancer a short time previously. She had a tumour "the size of a small water melon" and was told that it was likely that her bowel and stomach were also affected by the cancer. She had been prescribed chemotherapy "to try and prolong what life I had left". There were no guarantees of an operation. She said that "her world was collapsing around her".

In her own words: "The effects of having chemo and knowing I had cancer were awful. I was losing weight dramatically, constantly being sick, experiencing frequent incontinence, losing hair in large clumps and being in constant indescribable pain. I was practically the walking dead and at this point would have welcomed being put out of my misery."

Margaret said that she did not believe in complementary therapies or support groups, but she was willing to try anything. Her nurse had suggested that she dropped into the Centre to see what it was like and that if she didn't like it she could leave of her own accord. On arriving at the Centre, Margaret was relieved to see that "people were walking around, talking, being sociable and kind. It all made me feel like there was some hope. There were other women in similar if not possibly worse situations than me. I quickly realised that this was not a place of sickness but of hope."

During the course of her first visit, Margaret was shown around the Centre, offered refreshment, introduced to volunteers and clients and then was given the opportunity to talk to a therapist. The therapist listened as Margaret talked about the issues she and her family were experiencing due to the sudden diagnosis of cancer. She found this very helpful. The therapist also recorded information about Margaret's diagnosis, treatment and the problems she was experiencing and talked with Margaret about the therapies which she might find helpful. Over the next few weeks

Margaret had appointments for hypnotherapy, aromatherapy massage and homeopathy.

At that time the Centre was taking part in a national study programme to ascertain the effects of hypnotherapy with cancer patients including those undergoing chemotherapy. One of the Centre's hypnotherapists had attended a course on the methods of hypnotherapy required for the study which included some cognitive behaviour therapy (CBT) training and the Centre became a participating body in the study.

The hypnotherapist taught Margaret how to use her own mind to enhance the effects of the chemotherapy by using creative visualisation. This involved visualising the chemotherapy attacking the cancer cells using Margaret's own thought creations. Margaret was given an audio tape to help her with the visualisation and also a tape to aid relaxation. She listened to these every day and even took them to the hospital with her. Margaret says: "This may sound unbelievable to those of you reading this, but trust me, I had also been in the same frame of mind, but the programme really did yield amazing results. The more hypnotherapy I received the better I felt, both physically and emotionally. The sessions were reinforced with methods of self meditation which helped with my general well being and which I still use today."

Alongside the hypnotherapy sessions, Margaret was also receiving aromatherapy massages, which were gentle at first, but later the massage was deepened which helped Margaret to feel re-energised and aided de-stressing and relaxation. She also enjoyed Indian head massage.

The homoeopath provided Margaret with remedies to help her sleep better, to combat sickness and constipation and to improve her general well-being.

The combination of these therapies resulted in Margaret quickly starting to feel much better and enabled her to think more positively. The Centre became increasingly more important to her, not only as a place where she received therapies but where she met with other clients at the Thursday support group. It was a place where she could get physical and mental relief and also share her thoughts and concerns with support group members.

Margaret's improving well-being also relieved her family of the stress they had been feeling.

After 5 months of chemotherapy and complementary therapies received at the Centre, the doctors recognised Margaret's improvement and following a test showing that the tumour had shrunk in size, decided to operate. Not only did Margaret come through the operation, (she had been warned about possible complications), but the doctors were amazed that the cancer had not spread to other areas of the body and that somehow the tumour had effectively dissipated to little more than a "mush".

Margaret had more chemotherapy after the surgery which resulted in side effects as before, but continuing with complementary therapies aided her recovery and in a few months she was back to her old self. Effectively her cancer had disappeared.

Over the next couple of years Margaret continued to attend the support group, often offering a listening ear to other clients. She also attended some of the educational talks offered at the Centre. Many clients were interested in changing their eating habits to enhance their recovery. Margaret, however, was very conservative in her eating habits and had a dislike for many of the fruits and vegetables that were recommended. Over a period of time she found she could incorporate the vegetables she did not like into soups. A number of the clients used to bring tasters of the soups they had made, for her to try, which she did, sometimes with distaste.

Margaret also joined the walking group which did a few miles in Sutton Park once week. Another activity she was very fond of was dancing, so whenever there was a fund raising event such as a ball or a disco, Margaret and her husband would always be there having a great time.

For more than 3 years now, Margaret has been a volunteer at the Centre, acting as a receptionist once a week and at the same time talking to new clients and giving them hope for the future. She also does administrative work for her husband. It is now 5 years since Margaret had her operation and all her check ups have been positive. Margaret's son has helped the Centre with its web-site and leaflet production. He added his own comment to others on the leaflet: "Without the Centre's close support, I really don't think my mom would be here today. Thank you"

Margaret's feelings about the Centre are: "The therapists and volunteers made me feel like I was the only person being cared for. Even though that is not true, that is the feeling that they gave to each and everyone of us. I felt like I was in the safest hands in the world, and through the difficult times that I was going to be OK. If the Centre had not provided me with these wonderful people helping me and my family to cope with cancer, I really believe, I would not be here today. To say thank you is too little a word. I pray that the Centre can continue with its wonderful work. My family and I are forever indebted to the Centre".

Introduction to Therapeutic Activities at the Centre

The philosophy of the Centre (see below) was agreed soon after its inception and has remained the same since then. The fundamental belief is that healing needs to be holistic i.e. it involves body, mind and spirit. Also vital, is access to relevant information, empowerment, and the opportunity for choice.

The connection between body and mind may be obvious: one cannot work without the other, as each one transfers information to the other. However, there may be less understanding of the spiritual dimension of healing. Those who practice a particular religion may recognise the part spirituality plays in their healing but many believe that you can be spiritual without being religious. For example, some people believe that nature offers any number of spiritual experiences. Others experience sensations or emotions that convince them of their own spirituality. If we have spiritual experiences then we must be spiritual beings. If spirit is an integral part of each one of us the spirit needs to be healed, alongside body and mind, when we have been damaged by disease, surgery or traumatic events.

Most of those who practice and attend the Cancer Support Centre have a belief in spirituality but how they experience and express spirituality may differ considerably. The many therapies and activities provided at the Centre will offer an element of healing which may be considered spiritual. Clients may select therapies which complement their own particular spiritual beliefs.

The Centre does not have allegiance to any particular religion: its philosophy is to accept people from any background or belief system and work with those people to maximise their healing in a way that suits them.

The number of therapeutic techniques offered at the Centre has gradually increased during the last 10 years so that currently 12 individual therapies are available at the Centre as well as a range of therapeutic group activities.

The first therapeutic methods to be used were relaxation and creative visualisation. These were practiced in small groups and with individuals and led by trained counsellors and hypnotherapists. Individual counselling and hypnotherapy sessions were introduced as soon as rooms were acquired in which to run regular sessions. The belief in the value and power of relaxation and creative visualisation techniques has increased over the years as clients have demonstrated how well they worked for them. Recently the Centre has developed a relationship with Dr David Hamilton, whose book, "How Your Mind Can Heal Your Body", emphasises the power of creative visualisation and quotes evidence from many research projects. David has visited the Centre recently and is now offering workshops for clients and therapists there.

Philosophy

We Believe that:

- When a person is experiencing a disease, the effects are physical, psychological, emotional and spiritual
- Recovery involves attending to the needs of the whole person – body, mind and spirit
- Therapies which complement medical treatment can aid recovery and lessen the distressing symptoms that may occur as a result of the disease
- Family members and close friends of the person who has a physical disease may be suffering physically, psychologically, emotionally or spiritually as a result of their loved one's disease and will benefit from support and some of the therapeutic approaches we can offer
- Those experiencing disease will benefit from having the opportunity to make choices about their treatments and take some control in their lives
- Achieving a positive approach to the diagnosis of cancer will enhance the potential for recovery
- Therapies aimed at strengthening the immune system will enhance the potential for recovery
- Receiving a diagnosis of cancer can cause fear and vulnerability and therefore a gradual and gentle introduction to therapeutic ideologies is needed. Freedom of choice about treatments needs to be emphasised.
- Access to information is empowering.

For some time now, in addition to relaxation & creative visualisation classes, the Centre has offered weekly sessions of meditation. There is some similarity between the two but meditation sessions are usually longer and include slightly different techniques. Clients will try the different sessions and choose which suits them best. Some will attend both.

Reiki (energy) healing, various massage techniques and homoeopathy were offered at an early stage of the Centre's development as soon as therapists with appropriate skills offered their services.

The early popularity of Reiki healing led to the introduction of Reiki 1 training courses for clients and volunteers. This enabled those completing

11

the courses to use Reiki healing for their own benefit as well as offering it to close friends and family members. Many chose to continue with the Reiki 2 course so that they could use the skills learnt to benefit others. In fact a few clients, who learnt the skills at courses run at the Centre, are now practising therapists at the Centre. Reiki courses including the Masters' course are still offered regularly.

Courses which promote self-development and self-healing have been an important aspect of the therapeutic activities at the Centre throughout the last 10 years.

One of our first therapists was a trainer for "Heal Your Life" courses from Louise Hay, so this course was offered and proved to be successful. Later another Louise Hay trainer joined the team and the course continued to be offered regularly and proved to be very popular with clients. The Centre continues to offer courses based on the work of Louise Hay and now the work of David Hamilton and other authors is integrated into these courses.

Physical activity was always recognised as being part of the healing process, but in the early years, lack of space in the building being used meant that the Centre couldn't offer classes. However, as soon as larger premises were obtained, classes in Tai Chi, Qigong and Yoga were offered. Currently Yoga classes are offered weekly and are very popular.

A weekly walking group was started some years ago and continues still. The nearby, beautiful Sutton Park offers endless opportunities for different walks. Clients, therapists and volunteers also take part in the annual Great Midlands Fun Run which benefits them physically as well as helping to raise funds for the Centre. Our patron Sally Ellis, a past British Olympic marathon runner, offers training programmes for Fun Run participants.

Art classes have been offered for a number of years. These offer an opportunity to develop creative skills whilst having a relaxation effect.

Other creative and developmental activities which have been introduced include singing and a reading group. The singing group uses the new skills learned to sing carols and raise funds at Christmas time. At a recent Flower Festival lunch, our patron, Toni Christie, entertained the group by singing several of his popular numbers, including: 'Is This The Way to Amarillo'.

Talks and courses which promote healthy nutrition have also had a prominent place on the Centre's programme. Some clients choose to follow a dairy-free diet as promoted by Professor Jane Plant CBE, but client choice has always been the Centre's philosophy. Jane visited the Centre recently to give a talk and has subsequently become a patron of the charity. A previous client who became interested in nutrition and undertook training is now the nutritional advisor at the Centre.

Additional therapies offered in recent years are acupuncture, Bowen technique and Emotional Freedom Technique (EFT). EFT also offers the opportunity for self-healing as clients are taught a technique which they can then practise at home with very good effect.

Clients initially need to access therapies and therapeutic activities to manage their responses to a cancer diagnosis and to commence a holistic healing programme. Those affected by cancer may also bring with them a number of other physical, psychological and emotional issues which need to be addressed if holistic healing is to take place. The wide range of therapies available allows the Centre to offer therapies, which will address these additional issues, and also alleviate the side effects of treatment for cancer and other pre-existing physical problems.

Every new client is offered a preliminary consultation with a trained assessor so that their therapeutic needs can be assessed. When deciding on the therapeutic plan, the client is informed about suitable therapies and groups and then makes a choice of up to two individual therapies if required. Assessors have attended study days about the different therapies and have information files in order to help the clients make decisions about the most appropriate therapies for them. The number of therapies the client receives in total will be assessed according to client need. Clients can attend any group activity as long as there are spaces available. Clients are encouraged to participate in group activities and to attend talks and discussions as these contribute to the holistic healing programme.

The assessment process collects information from the client about their illness, previous and coexisting illnesses and medications. This information will help therapists to decide how they treat the client. For some therapies there may be some contraindications to giving the therapy and therapists will always check with the client when they attend for treatment if any of these are present.

After receiving a set number of individual therapies, a review consultation takes place to discuss the effect of the therapeutic plan and any future treatments the client might need. The Centre aims to look at each individual's needs when preparing a therapeutic plan and the needs may change as the client heals and progresses.

The holistic healing offered by the Centre depends on the commitment of therapists and group leaders, volunteers and staff who often offer more than is reasonably expected of them. A very caring atmosphere is generated at the Centre by all those who work there and I would venture to suggest that there is an element of love in the delivery of the service which has a very positive effect on the client's wellbeing. The clients themselves seem to react to this atmosphere of love and caring by showing care and love for the other clients they meet there and this in turn results in promoting holistic healing.

A Testimonial from a Client

I was so lucky to have found the Cancer Support Centre just before my bowel cancer operation. The warmth of the welcome and the kindness of staff and therapists were so comforting and encouraging. They straight away gave me therapies on a day the Centre is normally closed and also made me a relaxation tape to take into hospital, which meant I felt supported and found it easier to help in my own recovery.

In the following months I had therapies like Reiki, hypnotherapy, counselling. meditation and Bowen Technique which, together with courses and group discussions with other clients taught me a lot about changes I needed to make in my life. The books borrowed from the Library have meant I could look more deeply into new ideas.

I really think everybody touched by cancer can find something to help them at the Centre and in an atmosphere that is always cheerful and friendly.

References:

Louise Hay.	2009.	You Can Heal Your Life, Hay House UK
	2004	The Power Is Within You, Hay House UK
Dr David Hamilton.	2008	How Your Mind Can Heal Your Body Hay House UK
	2010	Why Kindness Is Good For You Hay House UK
Professor Jane Plant.	2000	Your Life in Your Hands, Virgin
	2004	The Plant Programme, Virgin
	2010	Eating For Better Health, Virgin

Self-Healing Activities

Relaxation, Creative Visualisation and Meditation

These therapeutic approaches have been taught and used at the Cancer Support Centre since its inception and have been valued by many as means of reducing stress and enhancing well being and healing. Although there are links between the methods and they all induce altered states of mind, each one will be explained separately to facilitate the reader's understanding of each and the special part they play in encouraging holistic healing. Scripts for relaxation, creative visualisation and meditation are included; these will help to illustrate the links.

Evidence from the scientific research of other authors supports the value of relaxation and creative visualisation and meditation. These are detailed in Your Mind Can Heal Your Body by Dr David Hamilton. The Centre offers group 'Relaxation' sessions, which include visualisation, and longer 'Meditation' sessions. Some therapists will also offer individual relaxation and visualisation to clients.

These techniques are valuable as aids to healing but they can also be of benefit to all human beings in reducing stress and enhancing wellbeing. Understanding of the value of these techniques as an aid to healing at the Centre has increased over the years.

Relaxation

There are numerous relaxation techniques that can be used; they will have the effect of relaxing the body and the mind as there is an inseparable link between the two. The body constantly transmits messages to the mind and the mind constantly communicates with the body. The acknowledgement of this body mind connection is vital in the delivery of all healing therapies and techniques.

Some relaxation techniques focus largely on relaxing parts of the body but as stated above the effect will be also to calm the mind. An example here is progressive muscular relaxation where groups of muscle are tensed and relaxed in order until the whole body is relaxed (See script below).

Another simple method of achieving relaxation is by focussing on the breathing. When we are anxious or stressed we take incomplete, frequent, shallow breaths, so we need to focus on breathing slowly and deeply in order to fill our lungs with oxygen but also to facilitate a more relaxed way of being. Even though anxiety and stress are created in the mind, by altering a physical activity such as breathing, the mind can be calmed. To breathe deeply, it is necessary to fully expand the lungs; this involves the lowering of the diaphragm and the widening of the rib cage. When you breathe like this you will be able to feel the rising of the abdominal wall as the diaphragm flattens. When we change the pattern of our breathing to slower and deeper breaths, this has the effect of calming the mind. Focussing on a few deep breaths is commonly used at the beginning of many relaxation and meditation techniques. Taking 3 or 4 deep breaths can induce relaxation in a stressful situation, so the technique is taught to anyone who experiences anxiety or anger suddenly.

Progressive Muscular Relaxation Technique

- Find a quiet, peaceful room and ensure that you will not be disturbed
- Sit or lie in a comfortable position
- Begin by focussing on your feet. Then curl your toes under and tense all the muscles in your feet. Hold this tension for a few seconds and then let go of the tension.
- Now focus on your knees and thighs, clench the knees together and tighten the muscles in your thighs. Hold for a few seconds and then release.
- Next focus on your buttocks and clench them together tightly. Hold the tension for a few seconds and then relax the muscles.
- Tighten the abdominal muscles, drawing your umbilicus towards your spine. Hold for a few seconds and then release.
- Focus on your hands and arms, clench your fists and tense the muscles in the arms drawing them close to the body. Hold for a few seconds and then let go.
- Pull your shoulders up towards your ears. Hold for a few seconds and then lower the shoulders down to a relaxed position
- Now tighten all the muscles in your face making a funny expression. Let go after a few seconds.
- Finish with a big yawn, then release all the facial muscles.
- Now experience and enjoy the relaxed feelings in the whole of your body for as long as you wish

Breathing Focussed Relaxation/Meditation Technique

- Find a quiet, peaceful environment where you will not be disturbed.
- Sit or lie in a comfortable position.
- Take a deep breath in (through your nose if possible), and concentrate on letting the air reach the bottoms of your lungs and letting your abdomen rise as this happens. Placing your hands, with finger tips touching, on your abdomen will allow you to experience the abdomen rising and the fingers parting. Hold the breath for a count of four and let the breath out slowly through your mouth or nose, allowing your abdomen to fall as the lungs empty and experiencing a sense of relaxation as you breathe out.
- Take two more deep breathes as above, feeling increasingly relaxed as you let go of the breaths.

- Now allow your breathing to settle into a more natural rhythm but still allowing the lungs to fill completely. Notice a deepening of the relaxation feelings every time you breathe out.
- You can continue to focus on your in and out breaths, increasing the level of relaxation, for as long as you wish or you may choose at this stage to follow with a creative visualisation.

NB A popular form of meditation involves focussing on the in and out breath and letting thoughts drift away

Creative Visualisation (Imagery)

Creative Visualisation is another common relaxation technique. It is used on many commercially available tapes and CDs. Here the focus is on using the mind to create positive images to promote a feeling of wellbeing which calms the mind and body. As the mind focuses on creating these images, other intruding thoughts gradually decrease.

Although this method is commonly called creative visualisation, it is important to recognise that vision is only one of the human senses and the other senses can also be used to deepen the experience, for example whilst visualising a beautiful scene, you can also employ the sense of hearing to listen to associated sounds, or skin sensation to recognise touch, warmth or cold. The senses of taste and smell can also be utilised. Some people do not have vision as their dominant sense and, if this is the case, it is important to explore using the other senses.

In some visualisations, there may be a focus on the chakras. Ancient philosophers believed in an energy system within the body consisting of seven major chakras or vortices which are like spinning wheels of energy situated throughout the head and trunk. These chakras are used by a number of complementary therapists, especially Reiki practitioners. The seven major chakras are identified by position and colours. The colours are related to the frequency at which the chakras vibrate.

According to ancient beliefs, there are also minor chakras in other parts of the body. Reiki practitioners believe that there are universal sources of energy outside the human body to which it is connected. Visualisation may include the taking into the body of energy and light through the chakra system.

CHAKRA	LOCATION	COLOUR
Crown	Top of Head	Violet
Brow or Third Eye	Centre of Forehead	Indigo
Throat	Throat	Blue
Heart	Centre of Chest	Green
Solar Plexus	Upper Abdomen	Yellow
Sacral	Abdomen/Navel	Orange
Base	Bottom of Spine	Red

Relaxation and creative visualisation used regularly can reduce blood pressure and decrease the heart rate, improve breathing so that the body's systems are better oxygenated and stimulate healing by improving immune system functioning. Stress and anxiety lower immune system activity but this effect can be reduced by the use of relaxation and meditation techniques.

<u>Comments made by clients who attend Relaxation groups:</u>

"I find relaxation calming; it helps me to deal with everyday stresses. I find I can cope better"

"The wonderful thing about relaxation is for a short time it is all about you. I leave feeling calm and ready for everything that life throws at me".

"It is the one chance to feel completely free of having to concentrate on all the things you need to be doing. Thoughts come and go, and the soft music and soothing voice leave you feeling great for the day ahead".

<u>Relaxation and Creative Visualisation to Promote Health</u>

Before following suggestions below, ensure that you are in a comfortable and safe place and that you will not be disturbed or interrupted for a period of at least 15 minutes.

- You can sit with your body well supported or you can lie flat. If you need to refer to this script, it may be better if you are sitting, but as you become familiar with it you may choose to lie down.
- Close your eyes if you feel comfortable to do so, but this is not always necessary and you may still need to refer to the script.

- Take 3 deep breaths, ensuring that you completely fill your lungs so that your stomach rises and letting the breath out slowly. Ideally breath in through your nose and out through your mouth
- With each slow breath out, experience a feeling of relaxation spreading through your body.
- Continue to breathe in and out slowly and experience the feeling of relaxation increasing and deepening
- Focus on your breathing and the relaxation experience and let other thoughts that might come into your mind float away
- As you become more relaxed, focus on any parts of your body which may not be totally well and visualise the relaxation feelings going to those parts and relaxing them
- If you find visualisation difficult you may want to focus on the sensations in those parts especially feelings of relaxation moving there
- Now let your mind focus on the wonderful abilities of your body to heal itself, the functions of the immune system and all the healing cells and substances it produces
- You can ask your immune system to increase its work to meet your needs
- Now, perhaps, you can sense the immune system increasing its activities and visualise the healing cells and substances going to the places where they are needed. You may be able to see or feel the blood moving through the vessels to deliver immune substances to the parts where they are needed. You may also be able to see or sense the toxins and waste materials being removed from the site. You can visualise or sense this in any way you choose e.g. a train or truck delivering the immune substances or a waterfall flushing away the toxins. Use your creative mind to create the best visualisations or sensations for you.
- Continue to practise these visualisations and sensations for a little while and then return to focussing on your breathing and becoming aware of every part of you body
- You can then start to move your limbs and open your eyes, when you are ready, telling yourself that you are now fully awake and alert and ready to carry on with your daily activities

Meditation

Meditation has much in common with other relaxation techniques and may often be seen as the same as relaxation, but there are some different ways of achieving this state of mind. Usually the person practising meditation will focus continuously on an activity or a word or a sound and this gradually results in the cessation of intruding thoughts. The aim is to accept intruding thoughts and let them go and then gradually these thoughts will stop intruding.

One simple method of meditating is to focus constantly on the breath coming and going. Several deep breaths may be taken at first and then a natural breathing rhythm achieved. Another method is to focus the eyes on a candle flame or a beautiful object placed a short distance away at eye level.

Some people who learn meditation will be given a mantra, a simple word or phrase, which they constantly repeat in their head to achieve the meditative state. Alternatively, a sound such as "ohm" can be sung or can reverberate in the head and become the focus of attention.

The meditation sessions at the Centre combine breathing techniques, relaxation of muscle groups and visualisation, but also focus on the chakras and the energies present in the universe and in the earth's core. Music used during these sessions is from the Buddhist tradition including the "ohm" sound and there is a period of silence as the desired state is achieved.

Comments from clients who attend Meditation sessions

"I have felt at peace and energised"
"The difference on leaving is wonderful. I feel so relaxed".
"It helps me to remain positive and happy"
"Meditation at the centre for me is:-
+ a time for peace and calm,
+ a time when I can find some space for me,
+ a time to let go of the physical world and explore the spiritual world,
+ a time to release emotional and mental constraints,
+ a time to be.

At the end of meditation I feel physically and mentally relaxed, calm, energised and prepared for the rest of the day and sometimes for the rest of the week".

Colour Meditation

- You can use the progressive muscular relaxation or the breathing technique to achieve a relaxed state.
- When you are feeling pleasantly relaxed, imagine yourself standing in the countryside looking at a fantastic rainbow in the sky.
- Focus your attention on all the colours: red, orange, yellow, green, blue, indigo and violet.
- Now you can begin to experience each colour separately.
- As you concentrate on red, allow your mind to make associations with the colour; perhaps you will see or smell red roses, or strawberries. Here you might also get a sense of taste. If the colour red represents any negative feelings for you, breathe deeply and focus on releasing these emotions like red balloons floating away through the air. Then continue to focus on positive associations. Enjoy the colour red.
- Next focus on orange and enjoy any positive associations with the colour such as fruits and flowers. Perhaps you can smell or taste these. Enjoy the colour orange.
- Now concentrate on the colour yellow and again make positive associations with the colour, perhaps a field of rape seed, buttercups or corn, or golden sands on a beach. Enjoy the colour yellow.
- Now turn your attention to green and its positive connections; green lawns, new shoots and leaves unfurling on trees in spring. Enjoy the colour green.
- And now, focus on the colour blue. You might imagine yourself walking through bluebell woods, beside a brilliant blue sea or looking up at a clear blue sky. Enjoy the colour blue.
- Focus next on the deeper blue, indigo and the associations that colour brings to mind, perhaps an item of favourite clothing or furnishings, or a night sky. Enjoy the colour indigo.
- Finally focus on the colour purple with its healing associations. See yourself walking in fields of lavender and breathe in the perfume. Spend as long as you wish enjoying the colour purple.
- When you are ready, see again the whole rainbow and spend a moment or two marvelling at its beauty, before slowly bringing yourself back to your quiet and peaceful place.

Reference

Dr David Hamilton.   2008   How Your Mind Can Heal Your Body
Hay House UK

Heal Your Life Course

The 'Heal Your Life' courses run at the Centre are based largely on the philosophy of Louise Hay with the premise that all human beings have the potential to heal themselves and that in order for self healing to occur there needs to be self love. This suggests that the absence of self love in many people's lives may be a factor in creating ill health. Also included in the course are philosophies based on the work of: Dr David Hamilton, Wayne Dyer, Bruce Lipton and Susan Jeffers.

A number of concepts are explored during the course. These include:

- Love
- Self love
- Fear
- Anger
- Relationships
- Forgiveness
- Work
- Abundance

Exploring some these concepts enables clients to consider the patterns in their own lives that may have contributed to their lack of self love, which may have played a part in the development of their illness.

Although these concepts are considered as foci, the individual clients and the group will in some ways direct the content and pace of the course. It is believed that the clients' needs are paramount and that the course belongs to them, although, the facilitator will direct and move the group along as necessary and ensure that the discussion is relevant to the course aims.

When addressing the need for self love, there are a number of exercises which are introduced. Perhaps the most important of these are 'Affirmations' and 'Mirror Work'.

Affirmations are positive messages that you say to yourself to increase your self love, for example "I love and accept you just the way you are". Looking into the mirror and looking into your own eyes as you say this makes the message all the more potent.

Prior to commencing these exercises there will have been ample opportunity to discuss the negative messages that each person has received throughout their lives. Using positive affirmations is a means of erasing these messages but as the negative messages have been repeated throughout a life time, affirmations need too be repeated daily throughout life in order to boost the self love and self esteem.

You might like to use the following affirmations or perhaps create your own. They will be more powerful if you can look at yourself in a mirror as you say them.

- I love and accept you just the way you are
- I am filled with love and affection
- I am joyous, happy and free

The negative messages that many receive throughout their lives will inevitably create fear and anger so these two emotions are explored fully during the course, enabling the clients to release negative feelings.

Another concept which is an important part of the course is forgiveness.

Learning to forgive is essential to feeling good about ourselves. When we forgive someone, we not only release that person but we also release ourselves from the anger, resentment and painful feelings we have been holding on to.

The course also addresses relationships, which are essential to human beings, but which also can cause distress and fuel feelings of low self worth. Changing the nature of a relationship or letting that relationship go can be important in self healing.

Two other interesting concepts are explored during the course: the law of attraction and abundance.

The law of attraction simply means like attracts like: if we think positive thoughts, we will attract positive things into our lives. Conversely when we think negative thoughts, we attract negative things into our lives.

With abundance, the belief is that the universe has a profusion of all that we may wish for. However, simply asking for what we want is not enough; in order for it to manifest we have to truly believe it will happen. The following affirmations may help you to manifest what you most want and need:

- I am slender
- I love my body
- I am prosperous
- I am totally healthy
- I trust the process of life will bring me to my highest good
- I deserve the best and accept it now

What Course Members have said about the Course.

"The Heal Your Life course has made a big impact on my life. I now feel my own self worth. I have far more peace. I do not listen to negative personal remarks. I use my affirmations all the time to remind myself how important I am. I do not allow other people to tell me how I should feel, think or act. I am learning every day; this will probably go on for the rest of my life. All my life I have felt inadequate. Not now!"

"It has made me feel a lot stronger. I look for the positive in life. I put myself first and live for the moment"

"I have felt a definite change in me and I will take a lot from the experience and use it in my everyday life. I am still on an important journey and whereas I was scared of finding out where I could end up, I now look forward with a new hope and anticipation."

"I shall be kind to myself and retain my power. I shall still enjoy being supportive to others but I will set my own boundaries without guilt."

References

Louise Hay.	2009	You Can Heal Your Life, Hay House UK
	2004	The Power Is Within You, Hay House UK
David Hamilton.	2008	How Your Mind Can Heal Your Body, Hay House UK

	2010	Why Kindness Is Good For You, Hay House UK
Bruce Lipton.	2005	The Biology Of Belief Mountain of Love/ Elite Books, Santa Rosa
Susan Jeffers.	2007	Feel The Fear And Do it Anyway, Vermillion

Lin's Story

In March 2004 I was diagnosed with Ductal Carcinoma in Situ (DCIS). Following my diagnosis, I was in total shock and disbelief, and although I didn't realise it at the time, my world had changed forever. It was not only my world that had changed, but my family's world too. Like many families, we didn't discuss this, but the impact on them must have been horrendously frightening. I too, can remember feeling frightened and very much alone.

Within two weeks, I had undergone major surgery. Although I felt an enormous trust for my consultant, which, I now know to be vital in the recovery from all illnesses, I sensed he was too busy to talk to me at any length during my follow up appointments. I knew that I needed to find local help and support; the hospital where I had my treatment was over ten miles away.

I took myself off to the breast cancer clinic at my local hospital and was advised to visit The Cancer Support Centre in Sutton Coldfield. This was to be one of the best pieces of advice I have been given in my life.

On arrival at the centre I was welcomed by the founder and then chairperson of the Centre. She immediately put me at ease; she told me about the ethos of the centre and introduced me to the volunteers who help to engender a sense of peace and calm. I was made to feel very special.

Following my initial assessment, I was offered a range of complementary therapies. Each one of these was given by a caring, sensitive and, professional therapist. I found the experience of receiving therapies such as Reiki, aromatherapy and reflexology very relaxing and invaluable to my healing both mentally and physically. I felt nurtured. I began to learn how to relax and was able to meet other people whose lives had been affected by cancer.

I also received invaluable help and support through counselling. Talking to a counsellor enabled me to talk openly about my fears and my experience of cancer. During the counselling sessions I was able to explore other traumatic times in my life. I became aware how these traumas may have played a part in my illness. I realised it was time to change my life. I felt a weight had been lifted off my shoulders as I released the hurt and pain that I had carried for most of my life. Being able to talk to someone in a non-judgemental and confidential environment definitely helped my mental health and wellbeing; in fact, I now believe that everyone would benefit from talking to a counsellor.

The Support Centre became (and still is) my sanctuary. For me, having cancer was the best thing that could have happened to me; by this I mean the illness gave me an opportunity to reflect on my life and to consider the factors that helped to create my illness.

I was able to participate in a number of personal growth and development workshops at the Centre. It has been through participating in these courses and my own personal therapy that I began to develop an understanding of who I AM. I have learned the importance of the power of the mind and how positive thoughts can help to heal the body. In addition, I have been able to discuss my diet with the nutritional advisor at the Centre and now eat the types of food that help to promote a healthy body. I also undertook Reiki training at the Centre and eventually became a Reiki master. I can now use those skills to help myself, clients at the Centre and those in my personal life.

I felt so deeply indebted to the therapists and clients at the centre that I felt I wanted to give something back, so in order to enable me to train to become a counsellor, I decided to resign from a teaching career. Now, I am able to offer help to those whose lives have been affected by cancer, both clients and their families. I am also leading courses based on the works of Louise Hay (You Can Heal Your Life), Dr David Hamilton (How Your Mind Can Heal Your Body) and others.

I know that by being at the Support Centre both as a client and now as a counsellor and group leader, I have been able to make positive changes in my life and have made many new friends, especially through attending the weekly group activities such as yoga and meditation.

I would like to thank everyone at the Centre for helping me to grow in mind body and spirit, essential ingredients I believe for my health and well-being.

Psychological Therapies

Counselling

Counselling is to an opportunity for clients to talk about aspects of their lives which are causing them distress. They will be able to talk about how they are feeling and explore areas and issues in their lives that they would like to change. The counsellor's role is to provide a supportive environment for the client and to listen to and validate the client's feelings. Although, the counsellor's role is not to give advice, they will be able to help the client to explore ways of achieving any changes they want to make in their lives.

There are many different models of counselling. Some counsellors may study one theory in depth and use that method only e.g. Cognitive Behaviour therapy or Gestalt therapy. Other counsellors will have studied numerous theories of counselling and methods of working with clients, which they adapt and utilise to meet each client's individual needs (Integrative counsellors). Whichever methods of counselling are used, the formation of a trusting relationship between client and counsellor is paramount.

Most clients who come to the Cancer Support Centre will be affected to some degree by loss or bereavement e.g. loss of body part or loss of independence and there are many theories and strategies which apply here. However, the primary function of the counsellor at the early stages of counselling is to listen and accept the client's story and its associated feelings.

As well as being affected to a greater or lesser extent by feelings of loss or grief, some clients also carry with them many other issues from their lives that may exacerbate these feelings of loss. It is therefore important that the counsellor is able to recognise these other factors and, if the client wishes this, incorporate them into the counselling process.

Counselling may be offered if clients talk about or show signs of anxiety, stress, fears, phobias, relationship problems, depression. These may be directly related to cancer and the loss situation or be a result of other factors in their lives. In order to contribute to holistic healing, the aim of counselling must be to help the client to resolve these difficulties. Of course, this aim needs to be the client's aim also.

As stress is generally accepted to be a factor in the development of cancers, anyone experiencing stress, anxiety, phobias, relationship problems or depression would benefit from counselling to overcome these problems as part of a healthy living programme. The holistic healing offered at The Cancer Support Centre is aimed at enhancing recovery from a cancerous disease but also at preventing reoccurrence.

Counsellors at the Centre generally work in what is usually termed a 'humanistic way', that is, they believe that the client 'knows best' and that all human beings have the capacity for change and for personal growth. Therefore counselling is not directed by the counsellor, it is the client who sets the agenda for the counselling work. The focus is on facilitating clients to find their own strategies for change. Confidentiality is a crucial aspect of all counselling and is discussed with clients at the beginning of the relationship.

Referral for counselling at the Centre is usually made by the person who conducts the initial assessment of the client or it could be the through one of the other therapists who is delivering a different therapy, such as Reiki or aromatherapy. If it is considered that counselling may be of benefit to a client, this is explored with them and if agreed, an appointment for a preliminary counselling session is made.

Hypnotherapy

Hypnosis is a natural state of relaxation during which the conscious mind becomes less active and the subconscious mind becomes more accessible. When clients are in this state of relaxation the body's systems can function more effectively and they can become more aware of the activities in their bodies and direct their own healing. The suppression of the conscious mind allows them to disconnect from worries and concerns and learn how to live life in a more fulfilling way. Sometimes, concerns that they have held in the subconscious mind for a long time, can be released.

Hypnotherapists need to talk with clients to ascertain the concerns they have which could be helped by hypnosis. They also need to carefully explain how hypnosis works and what the clients might achieve through hypnosis. Clients need to be aware that when they are in a hypnotic trance, they are still in control and can bring themselves out of that trance state whenever they wish. It is also helpful to explain the natural trance state which the hypnotherapist will assist them to achieve. This state of mind often occurs spontaneously in everyday life, for example when daydreaming or when absorbed in a book or a film. Before the hypnotherapist induces a hypnotic trance, the client needs to give permission for this to happen. The client needs to know that hypnotherapists are members of professional organisations, work to a code of ethics and offer clients confidentiality.

Hypnosis can be used to resolve any number of physical and emotional problems. Examples here are: chronic pain, low self esteem, lack of confidence. It can also be used to work with addictions such as smoking.

Hypnotherapy has special purposes when working with those who have cancer: For those clients who are having chemotherapy treatment, hypnotherapy can assist in overcoming needle phobias, increasing vein size to facilitate the insertion of needles and in raising blood counts to levels which are acceptable for treatment to take place.

For all those with cancer, visualisation can be used with hypnosis so that the client can see/sense cancer cells being removed from the body and healing taking place. The hypnotherapist can help clients to develop their own personal visualisations which will work for them. These visualisations can also be used with the aim of increasing the effects of chemotherapy or radiotherapy on cancer cells.

Clients can be taught self-hypnosis so that they can carry on working on themselves in between therapy sessions and after the therapy has finished, giving the client a greater sense of control over their wellbeing.

Clients who come to the Centre do not only bring their cancer diagnosis. Often they bring other concerns and emotions which hypnosis can benefit.

Hypnosis is particularly effective with phobias and post traumatic stress syndromes. It is not unusual to discover that clients who present with a cancerous disease have experienced traumatic events and sometimes abuse earlier in their lives and the feelings attached to these events still affect them. In order for these clients to heal well from their cancer, they need to release these feelings and develop a new perspective of their lives. Hypnotherapeutic techniques can be of great help here.

Hypnotherapy can aid clients to change the way they think and perceive things and as feelings follow thoughts, feelings are changed too. Many hypnotherapists are also trained in NLP (Neuro-linquistic Programming) and integrate these techniques into their work. This involves training the brain to think differently. Of course, the hypnotherapist will only help the client to change the thinking patterns which the client wishes to change. A general example here might be to change the clients' thinking about smoking so that it is no longer attractive and compelling to them. When a client has cancer, thought change could be related to how the client views hospitals, surgery and injections, so that treatment is completed with less anxiety and pain. Specific examples here are fear of needles, anaesthetic and hospitals in general.

Sometimes, clients have fears about needles, anaesthetics and hospitals which may have been triggered by one or more events in their early lives. Hypnotherapy techniques can help these clients to change their thinking and feelings about these events so that their fears are removed or reduced.

When working with fears and phobias, hypnotherapists will be aware that it is sometimes not appropriate to remove the fear completely, for example for people with fears of heights or deep water; they need to enable clients to retain a sufficient concern for those phenomena to ensure their own health and safety.

Hypnotherapists use relaxation techniques in order to induce a hypnotic trance and creative visualisation will often be included to aid deepening of the trance. Creative visualisation is also an important part of the therapy when working with clients who have cancer, using the visualisations to bring about changes in thoughts, feelings or behaviours in order to heal the body and mind. Margaret's story illustrates how hypnotherapy can assist in holistic healing.

Emotional Freedom Technique

Emotional Freedom Technique (EFT) is based on the theory that the cause of all negative emotions is a disruption in the body's energy system. Every time we experience an emotion, the body's energy system is influenced. EFT has been specifically designed to directly interact with the energy system, to enable our energy to flow freely again. EFT can address any and all situations that provoke an emotional reaction.

The practice of EFT involves tapping with the finger tips to stimulate certain meridian positions on the head, face, hands and upper torso, as the client focuses on 'the problem' or negative emotions they are experiencing. The meridians are the energetic pathways within the body that relay information to the entire system. These meridian points are also used in acupuncture and so EFT is sometimes referred to as acupuncture without needles. EFT works to realign the disrupted energy meridians and address underlying negative emotions. It is very effective for victims of trauma and abuse, fears and phobias, anxiety and depression, panic attacks, addictions and compulsions, resulting in feelings of relaxation and peace. EFT is a gentle healer; relief is achieved with little or no pain. EFT practitioners will normally teach the client a tapping sequence they can use at home so that healing is achieved more quickly.

Many people can now comprehend that the mind can affect the body, but few people realize that it is a two way street, the body can also affect the mind. Tapping the meridian points on the body whilst focussing on an emotional difficulty can change thinking. Just tapping on certain meridian ending points can re-balance the energies of the body, releasing unwanted emotions allowing a sense of inner calm to return.

As well as being a spiritual and emotional healer, EFT effects relief for a wide range of physical symptoms including headache, pain and excess weight. It may be that physical symptoms disappear or begin to heal when underlying negative emotions are resolved. EFT is very simple but powerful. Problems from the past as well as the present and the future can be treated.

The Centre's EFT practitioner says:

"I have used this system extensively with cancer clients and have found it to be very useful. It gives the client something to do for themselves, as it is quick and easy to learn, which gives them a sense of participating in their own recovery.

As most of us realise, cancer doesn't just 'happen'; there are many emotions way back in time that have a long term effect on the mind and body. So, to be able to clear the 'clutter' of the mind is very helpful practice in enabling peoples' recovery from all manner of ills and phobias.

I would recommend it most highly for therapists to use alongside other therapies or in a stand alone capacity".

<u>An Example of how EFT has helped a Cancer Centre client:</u>

One young lady, a single mother with a family of three, whose mother had recently been diagnosed with terminal cancer, came to the Centre for help with coming to terms with her grief. She had sessions with a hypnotherapist who also practiced EFT. Part of her problem was a compulsion to clean her house, doing this at least 12 times a day. She was taught how to use EFT by the therapist and practised it regularly with the desired effect. Within a few weeks she was only cleaning her house once a day if at all. This young lady is now training to be a counsellor, having already undertaken courses in several other therapies.

Sally's Story

Sally was diagnosed with synovial sarcoma of the neck in 2005. For one year preceding the diagnosis, she had experienced unbearable pain in her neck. Sally consulted her GP and was referred to specialists who requested tests and an MRI scan but could not make a diagnosis. They prescribed numerous pain killing medications, cortisone injections to the shoulder joint and also Botox injections but nothing would stop the pain. The Botox made it difficult for Sally to move her head. Sally was becoming desperate. The only thing that would deaden the pain a little and help Sally to get some sleep was alcohol.

Finally, after Sally pointed out the lump in her neck, further scans were arranged. This time a tumour was seen and Sally had a biopsy of the tumour. The biopsy was one of Sally's most agonising experiences; the local anaesthetic did not control the nerve pain. From the biopsy, the diagnosis was made and surgery followed. Six weeks after surgery, radiotherapy was commenced and the side effects of this caused Sally great distress. She was unable to eat solid food and had noises in her ear. Then the intense headaches started. These could last for several minutes or more and at one time Sally was having these excruciating pains 80 -100 times a day. These were a result of damage to the brain caused by the radiotherapy. Fortunately now, almost 5 years later, these may only occur once or twice a day. During the worst times Sally was taking up to 34 tablets a day, some for pain relief and some to counteract the side effects of the pain killers. Some made her sleep for 18 hours a day and she would eat very little, others caused her be very hungry which meant that her weight fluctuated.

It was after Sally had completed her radiotherapy treatment that Sally's mum saw a piece in the local paper about The Cancer Support Centre and Sally came along to find out how she might be benefit from what the Centre has to offer.

Sally tried a number of the complementary therapies on offer and all provided some relief from her pain, anxiety and depression. These included Reiki, hypnotherapy, Bowen technique and reflexology. She also consulted the nutritional therapist. But it was acupuncture and counselling which helped her the most. Acupuncture helped by balancing her energies and reducing pain. Sally still has regular acupuncture sessions. Sally says it is "amazing".

In the last few years, Sally has experienced traumatic events in her personal life and at one point became extremely low. It was then that counselling proved to be a "life saver". The counsellor used various strategies including art therapy to enable Sally to come to terms with the changes in her life.

Sally has attended groups and events at the Centre over the years and has made many friends there which she has found tremendously supportive.

There were some high spots in the last few years. In 2007, Sally celebrated her 30th birthday and the donations from guests at the party were given to the Cancer Support Centre.

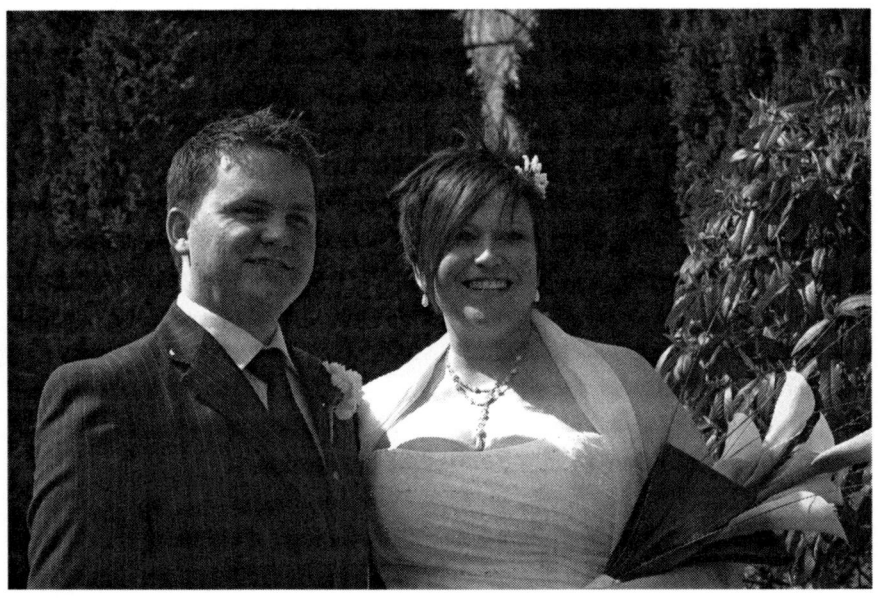

Sally & Steve on their Wedding Day

It was soon after this that Sally met Steve and started a relationship which led to their wedding in 2010. This was a wonderful occasion on a beautiful day and Sally looked so happy. A year or two before she could not have contemplated this could happen and she says that with out the counselling she would never had been able to make this commitment. Sally and Steve had a wonderful honeymoon in the Maldives and were planning to become foster parents, but, now to their surprise and joy they are expecting their own child in 2011.

Sally says "I could never repay the Centre for what they have done. Cancer is a very lonely disease. If people could come here, they would not be so lonely"

Energy Therapies

Reiki

Hands on healing of various kinds has been used in numerous societies throughout the world for thousands of years and today western societies have adopted a number of these. Reiki has become popular in the United Kingdom since the 1980's, although it was being practised in the United States long before this. It has its origins in Japan.

The word Reiki can be translated from the Japanese as "universal life force energy" or "divine-directed life force energy" or "spiritual energy". In the West, the form of Reiki practised is usually based on the healing practice of Dr Mikao Usui (1865–1926), a Japanese Buddhist priest. However, neither the giver nor the receiver needs to be a believer in a particular religion, only have faith in the 'universal life force energy'.

Ancient cultures of the world recognised that man and the universe are interconnected through an energy field. Modern science, especially Quantum Physics supports this belief. Human beings emit energy and can also absorb energy. This is the basis of Reiki. The Reiki practitioner absorbs energy from the universe and transmits it to the recipient. This energy taken into the body can have a healing effect on physical and emotional problems. During a Reiki session, a person may experience a deep feeling of relaxation and calm and afterwards may feel relief from physical symptoms. Reiki can be given in three ways, either "hands on", "hands off", or from a distance. The Reiki practitioner asks for the energy to given from the highest source he or she knows, and has the intention for the Reiki energy to be given for the highest good of the receiver. The hands are usually placed on or above the seven main chakras (energy centres of the body) during the course of a treatment.

Penelope Quest, Reiki For Life (2003) says "Reiki is not a guaranteed 'cure-all', because 'healing' is not always the same as 'curing'." and "Ultimately, if the healing is to be permanent you (the recipient) have to take responsibility for healing the cause. This may mean changing how you think or the way you relate to other people, or even altering your whole lifestyle, from your diet and home environment to your close relationships, your job or career.... there is really only one healer of your body, and that is you, because your body possesses the mechanisms to heal itself, so all anyone else can do - whether that person is a doctor, a nurse or a complementary therapist- is to kick-start that natural healing process in some way, whether by conventional or alternative means."

As Reiki becomes more popular in the West, different ways of practicing it will inevitably be developed. Penelope Quest says: "Reiki is a dynamic energy so it is bound to develop, and we will probably see even more 'versions' of Reiki in the future."

Reiki Training

Anyone can train to be a Reiki practitioner. There are three levels of training:

Reiki First Degree (Level 1)

This level is used for healing the self. During this level of training, the students learn to perform a full body treatment on themselves as well as learning the "hands on" positions for treating close friends and family. They also receive attunements from a Reiki master to re-awaken the energy centres in their hands, heart and third eye so that more universal energy can flow through the practitioner. First degree Reiki training has taken place at the Centre from early in the centre's history, so that those who wish to, can do self-healing.

Reiki Second Degree (Level 2)

At this level the students extend their knowledge of Reiki and are introduced to the Sanskrit symbols, which were rediscovered by Dr Usui, and also distant healing. They learn about the Chakras (energy centres in the body) and will receive further attunements. After this level of training, the students can start to practice Reiki on others, not just close friends and family, and can charge for these sessions if they wish.

Reiki Third Degree (Masters level)

Persons who have practised Reiki for a minimum of six months can study at this level. Only Reiki masters can teach levels 1 and 2 and give the required attunements.

A considerable number of clients at the Centre have learned Reiki over the years and some have progressed to Second degree and Masters Level. A few previous clients are now practising as Reiki practitioners at the Centre.

Reference:

Penelope Quest.   2002 Reiki For Life, Piatkus

The Centre's Reiki Master's Experiences and Thoughts

I was first introduced to Reiki in 1999. It sounded like a very interesting therapy to learn and would fit alongside the aromatherapy and reflexology that I was studying at college. I went to my first Reiki meeting and wondered what I had let myself in for. Everyone was talking about 'Energy' and feeling 'Energy' and connecting with 'Source.' At the end of the two hour lesson I thanked the teacher, who was a nursing sister at the local hospice, and said that I didn't think this Reiki thing was for me. She, my Reiki master, was however wiser than I and persuaded me to come back for another lesson and, as they say, the rest is history. I went on to qualify as a master myself in 2001 and then to teach Reiki. I think Reiki would be impossible to understand for a mind closed to spirituality.

Reiki is something everyone can do. It is a means of connecting with our inner self, our right brain person. It has its present day origins most probably in Buddhism but I rather suspect that its real origins go back to a period of time when the human species first became aware of its existence in the enormity of the universe. People in the past looked for a connection to all that was around them a link to the energy of the world in which they lived and they found that connection within themselves. By connecting to the energy of the universe they became aware of the energy within themselves and, aware of the energy of life, that runs through everything, and without which nothing exists.

Today science has revealed to us the enormity of the universe, the complexity of the galaxies, planets and stars, the existence of black holes and the unimaginable amount of space and energy that constitutes ours and other worlds. At the same time it has revealed the complexity of our own bodies, the inner workings of our cells, the story of DNA and the vast areas of space that exist within our cells. Science has also revealed that these vast areas of space contain waves of energy. In fact everything we see and encounter, whether it is animal, vegetable or mineral, it is made of energy. So Reiki is not very surprising after all, as it is the means by which we connect the energy of our body to that of the universe. It is our connection to the universal grid system or our connection to Source.

What Source is will depend on how we look at life as well as on our culture and upbringing. As Reiki is always given for 'the highest good and the greatest good' of the client, we should be able to assume that it is as safe as giving a prayer for someone. The energy of the universe is 'stepped down' to connect with the energy of this planet so that a safe amount of energy is given to the client. This energy will travel through the energy lines of the client's body, the meridian lines, helping to clear them of any blockages that may have been caused by stress, illness, or medication. Once this happens the client feels more relaxed, their energy lines start to become clearer and this will allow them to start their own healing process. Balance is the key to everything in this world and so the amount of energy Reiki can give will be proportional to how much negative debris needs to be cleared from our clients' bodies. If we have always smoked or taken drugs or alcohol in excess and continue to do so, then Reiki will have a more limited effect on helping us to feel well. If however we give ourselves Reiki or receive Reiki on a regular basis and start caring for our bodies, then we can enjoy the benefits of Reiki and feel healthier and calmer.

Reiki can be given to someone whilst they are sitting or lying down and there is no need to get undressed to receive it. It will work alongside other treatments and doesn't interfere with any tablets, chemotherapy or radiotherapy that the client may be receiving. The intent of Reiki is always to give 'love and healing' for the highest and greatest good of the recipient. A Reiki session usually takes up to an hour and is intended to be a form of deep relaxation, but Reiki can be given for just a few minutes as a first aid treatment if needed. It is widely used now, both in hospitals and hospices, where Reiki practitioners will have additional skills to enable them to work in these areas. There are several different types of Reiki qualifications but most practitioners working within the NHS or in similar areas will have Usui Reiki qualifications at Master level and will belong to a professional institute such as The Reiki Federation or The Reiki Association both of which have Codes of Ethics designed to protect clients.

I find that it is very empowering to learn Reiki and to be able to give yourself healing whenever you feel you need it. At the Cancer Support Centre we have always believed in trying to give clients and their families the tools to help themselves. We, the professionals, are always willing to give help but we are not always around when a person feels low or is in pain and it is at times like these that, by teaching them to give themselves Reiki, we are enabling them to help themselves. The Centre has always offered free Reiki Level 1 training for clients and their carers and we continue to run courses several times per year both at week-ends and in the evenings so that everyone who wants to learn has a chance to attend.

Some examples of the effects of Reiki

1. One of my very first students was a man with a high pressure job who learned Reiki with me and found that if he gave himself Reiki before a difficult meeting at work, it calmed him down and he was able to keep cool and focused throughout the meeting. He was using Reiki as a form of meditation to great effect and reducing the stress of his work.

2. A friend of mine, who was well into her 70's was diagnosed with bowel cancer and before her initial operation and treatment she learned Reiki with me. She would give herself healing on a regular basis and made a speedy recovery from the surgery much to the amazement of the nursing staff. Although she kept as well as possible for quite a few years, it eventually became apparent that her illness was progressing. As she became gradually more incapacitated I would visit on a regular basis and give her Reiki. I would concentrate on working over the inguinal lymph nodes of the groin to help reduce the possibility of the legs swelling, a condition known as lymphedema, which is caused by to the lymph nodes becoming increasingly damaged due to the spread of the cancer. She managed to stay free of lymphedema right up to the last few days of her life and she found that the Reiki gave her and her family tremendous ability to cope with her impending death.

3. I was fortunate enough to be able to give some Reiki to a young woman with a brain tumour. She would receive radiotherapy on a regular basis to try and shrink the tumour and I would try and give her Reiki the day following her treatment. She had never used holistic therapies before but she said that Reiki was the only thing that would help her brain to be 'unscrambled' after the radiotherapy.

I firmly believe that Reiki is not a miracle cure but I do believe that it helps you to be as well as possible at whatever stage of your life's journey. It helps you relax and allows your body to get on with the job it is designed to do- to look after you as best it can.

Quantum Touch

Quantum Touch (QT) is a method of hands-on healing that uses a very light touch to accelerate the body's own healing response (Gordon 2002). To use QT the therapist needs to learn various breathing techniques, body awareness, meditations and hand positions.

The ability to heal is an inherent part of our essential nature, as is our body's ability to heal itself: "A healer is a person who was sick and got well. A great healer is a person who was very sick and got well quickly"!

Quantum Touch (QT) was introduced at the Cancer Support Centre after a number of the therapists participated in a Basic QT Video Workshop in 2006. In order to become registered QT Practitioners, it is necessary to also attend a Live Basic QT workshop and purchase and read Richard Gordon's book: "Quantum Touch: The Power to Heal". It is also required that students document sixty hours of QT practice to be sent to the QT organisation in America, Two therapists attended the Live Workshop and progressed to QT Practitioner status. Practitioners sign up to a code of ethics and QT practice is included in existing professional insurance.

The beneficial effects for clients were apparent immediately after the video workshop, with one person's severe elbow pain alleviated with a 10 minute treatment. This gave the therapists the confidence to use the technique extensively for pain management.

Where QT fits in as Energy Therapy / Medicine: The diagnostic and therapeutic use of energy (Oschman 2003)

Vibrations underlie virtually all aspects of nature. In the living body each electron, atom, molecule, cell, tissue and organ and the body as a whole has its own vibratory character. Living structures and functions are orderly, biological oscillations and organised in meaningful ways. They contribute information to a dynamic vibratory network that extends throughout the body and into the space around it.

Dr Richard Gerber (1988) wrote that from an energetic standpoint, the human body when weakened oscillates at a different and less harmonious frequency than when healthy. If the individual is supplied with a dose of a much needed energetic frequency, it allows the cellular bio-energetic systems to resonate in the proper vibrational mode, thereby throwing off the illness.

Oschman states that the science of vibrations applies to all clinical methods, regardless of the techniques being used. Intricate energetic reactions occur between nearby individuals, even if they are not in direct contact. Information can be transferred from one organism to another via energy fields and living systems are very sensitive to them. Add therapeutic intention and touch to the equation and a whole new dimension of subtle but measurable exchanges are brought in to play.

Modern researchers have confirmed that living organisms do comprise dynamic energy systems involving the same sorts of Field phenomena that physicists have been studying for a long time.

Vibrational therapies are not magic; they are based on biology, chemistry and physics. It is through a series of vibratory energetic interactions that the various energy therapies have their effects.

It has been scientifically demonstrated that the energy field projected from the hands of body workers are in the range of intensity and frequency that can influence regulatory processes within the body of another person (Oschman P 135/6)

Example of a QT Treatment

- Discussion with client and assessment of need.
- Record severity of symptoms on Visual Analogue Scale before and after session.
- Focus on client, intend the client's wellbeing (Energy follows thought)
- Breaths: To hold a high vibration to which the client can entrain.
- Touch, hand positions, acknowledge body intelligence and chase the pain.
- Visualisations/meditations.
- Maintain dialogue with client. This is an interactive therapy.
- Relax and have fun with QT! "We know no limits with this work" (Gordon 2002)

In addition to being an effective pain management therapy Quantum Touch is also beneficial for general relaxation and the promotion of wellbeing

<u>Holistic Well-being Session:</u>

+ Assess and document client's need,
+ With client seated, balance Occipital Ridge, Atlas & Axis, C7 &T1 vertebrae, neck and hips.
+ With client on couch run energy in to both sides of head.
+ Work on major organs.
+ Work on endocrine system.
+ Treat lymphatic system especially head and neck, chest. axillary and groin nodes.
+ Work on any areas of concern/ disease.

Expected outcomes are muscular relaxation, stress reduction, pain relief, improved immune system and endocrine function, helping to align structural abnormalities and improve general health. (Gordon 2002)

<u>References</u>

Gerber R.	1998	Vibrational Medicine. Bear, Santa Fe. NM.
Gordon R.	2002	Quantum – Touch, The Power to Heal North Books USA.
Oschman J.L.	2003	Energy Medicine, The Scientific Basis. Churchill Livingstone, London

Reflexology

Many civilisations have practiced versions of reflexology for centuries. It is believed that the earliest form originated in China as much as 5000 years ago. It is possible that reflexology preceded acupuncture. A precursor to reflexology was introduced in the west in 1913 by William H. Fitzgerald, M.D. of the United States. He called this zone therapy.

Reflexology was further modified by Eunice D. Ingham (1889–1974), a nurse and physiotherapist. It was at this time that it was renamed reflexology.

Reflexology is based on the principle that there are reflex areas on the soles of the feet and the palms of the hands which correspond to all the body's structures, organs and glands. The therapist applies pressure with the fingers and thumbs to the reflex points on the feet and sometimes the hands. Normally the hands are only used if it is not possible to use the feet, although it is easier to give reflexology to oneself using the hands.

Reflexologists and other complementary therapists believe that blockages to the flow of energy (Qi) in the body can cause disease and that releasing these blockages to the energy flow, by the use of reflexology or other therapeutic techniques, can aid healing. Acupuncture is also based on this principle. The purpose of reflexology is, by using systematic application of pressure to the specific reflex points on the feet or hands, to relieve congestion, encourage the excretion of toxins, promote the flow of energy and encourage homoeostasis.

Reflexologists do not diagnose specific medical problems but when working on the reflex areas on the feet, the therapist can often identify possible problems and give attention to the specific related areas on the foot. The intention is to treat the individual holistically with a view to alleviating physical and emotional symptoms. When the client has cancer or is generally frail, only gentle pressure is applied.

Reflexology treatment is usually done with the client lying on a couch or a reclining chair. Often the therapist plays relaxing music during the treatment. There is no need to remove any clothing, only shoes and socks/tights. The treatment takes about 30 to 40 minutes.

Most people receiving a reflexology treatment find it very relaxing and this in itself can relieve stress and promote a feeling of well being. Reflexology is also known to relieve anxiety, pain, discomfort, constipation, insomnia and to stimulate healing. Clients are encouraged to drink plenty of water after a treatment to assist in the removal of toxins

There are a few contraindications to the use of reflexology, such as diseases of and injuries to the feet, but the therapist will make a full assessment of the client's medical situation before commencing a treatment.

One of the Centre's reflexologists reports that clients comment about how reflexology helps them to achieve a state of deep relaxation and that during the time of treatment they completely switch off from their daily tasks and concerns. Clients have also felt the energy moving through their bodies. They have also noted that any water retention in the feet and ankles is reduced quite significantly during a reflexology session. Some clients have also experienced pain reduction.

Reference

Ann Gillanders   1995   Reflexology: A Step By Step Guide,
                            Gaia Books

Eric's Story

In 2002, Eric, 79, and his wife came to the Cancer Centre for help and support in dealing with his diagnosis of cancer and their decision for him not to have any further medical treatment for this condition.

Eric had discovered a swelling in his neck which, after investigations and removal of one parotid gland, was found to be cancerous. The doctors noticed a further swelling on the opposite side of his neck which they also considered to be cancerous. Eric was offered radiotherapy to treat these swellings but having had the side effects of such treatment explained by the oncologist, he and his wife decided that, at his age, the side effects would seriously affect his quality of life, and so he turned down the treatment.

At the Cancer Centre, Eric and his wife were offered support and counselling to help them to come to terms with their decision and to make the most of the time they had left together. Eric was also offered Reiki healing, hypnotherapy and homoeopathy. These were integrated into a holistic programme of care. Eric and his wife also joined in some of the social activities at the Cancer Centre and attended meals out with other clients and volunteers at the centre. They also enjoyed the Annual Ball on several occasions. Eric and his wife also followed advice on healthy eating. Eric also found the prayers of his friends at the local Methodist church and another Christian group he attended to be of tremendous support.

Eric rarely suffered any pain or discomfort in his neck but had regular checkups with his GP and the hospital. Two years after his original diagnosis, Eric had a scan which reported that no sign of cancer could be found. The Centre has been given a copy of that result. After over two years of attending the Centre for treatment, Eric's general health remained good for an octogenarian and he and his wife were offered accommodation in another part of the country and made the move. The Centre had correspondence from Eric and his wife and 5 years after the original diagnosis Eric (aged 84) was still in generally good health.

Eric, his wife and therapists at the Centre believed that the holistic therapies he received contributed towards his continued health and the disappearance of the cancerous growths which were diagnosed. He also believed that the prayers of his Christian friends contributed to his continued wellbeing.

Massage Therapies

Aromatherapy

Aromatherapy is the use of essential oils most commonly applied by massage. The Essential Oils are wonderfully aromatic, and stimulate the sense of smell and an emotional response when used in aromatherapy.

Aromatherapy is a holistic remedy – affecting the mind, body and spirit, and is capable of promoting a sense of well-being. Massage used in conjunction with essential oils has many effects. There is the evocative power of the perfume of the oils used which can have an enhancing effect on our mood - smells are interpreted by the area of the brain concerned with our emotions.

The basis of the massage is touch – stroking, kneading, using light or deep pressure, rolling and loosening tight knotted muscles, relieving tension, improving circulation, and encouraging lymphatic drainage and the elimination of waste products. It may be relaxing or stimulating depending on the type of massage and the oils used.

Massage is not offered as an alternative to orthodox medical treatments. It is an antidote to the rigours of treatment, addressing the whole person rather than the diseased part.

Those newly diagnosed with cancer are likely to feel shocked, and the fear and tension associated with this may last for weeks. During this time of introspection and fear, breathing may be shallow with a possible tendency to hyperventilate. Muscles may contract, constricting the circulation of blood and lymph. This has a debilitating effect on the immune system at a time when it needs to work to its highest capacity. There is a need to feel safe, calm and protected to reverse this pattern.

The gentle, physical contact in aromatherapy is soothing and calming for the whole person. At a time when the relationship with professionals is focussed on the diseased part of the body' the contact between the massage practitioner and the person with cancer allows her/him to regain her/his view of herself as a whole and valued person. The gentle physical, non-invasive contact begins the process of acceptance of a changed body image.

Aromatherapy massage has a vital role to play in breaking the stress cycle of anxiety and insomnia which underlies so many physical complaints. Increasing evidence shows that stress affects not just the mind but also the nervous, immune and endocrine systems and constitutes a factor in both physical as well as mental health.

The Benefits of an Aromatherapy Massage.

- It provides a soothing and comforting alternative to verbal therapeutic techniques, such as counselling.
- It eases muscular aches and pains and promotes muscle relaxation and tone.
- It improves the circulation and lymphatic drainage, and helps to eliminate toxins from the body.
- It lowers blood pressure, reduces stress levels, and will help combat insomnia.
- It generates confidence and a feeling of well-being by releasing endorphins, the brain's natural opiates.
- It stimulates the immune system and strengthens resistance to disease.
- It aids digestion, eases constipation, and relieves abdominal spasm.
- Massage imparts a warmth and glow to the skin, and is revitalizing and rejuvenating to the whole body.
- It can alleviate tension headaches, and help the recipient to deal with difficult emotions, such as anxiety, depression, grief, or a sense of being unloved.

Aromatherapy Massage:

- Can improve the quality of life
- Aids relaxation
- Helps relieve stress, tension and anxiety

- Relieves symptoms of the disease and its treatment, both holistically and clinically
- Provides security and comfort through touch
- Gives empathy and time which is unhurried
- Uses a holistic approach whenever possible to evaluate each patient's needs
- Provides a one-to-one environment where patients can talk freely and in confidence.

Indian Head Massage (IHM)

Indian Head Massage (IHM) is a deeply relaxing treatment. It has been practised in India for centuries, with each family having their own massage techniques. Today in the western world a selection of these techniques has been put together to create a massage which helps to relieve tension in the shoulders, neck and head. Like many other massages, the therapeutic touch of IHM conveys feelings of warmth, relaxation and security. These are all beneficial to good health.

The treatment involves working in a firm and gentle way to manipulate the soft tissue of the shoulders, arms, neck, scalp, head and face. This treatment has proved successful at unblocking and relieving any uncomfortable build up of tension in these areas.

Whilst relieving muscle tension in the head, neck, shoulders, upper back and chest, IHM can improve the flow of blood and lymphatic circulation, which in turn increases the supply of oxygen to the brain. IHM has also been shown to be effective in helping to aid scalp and hair conditions.

This treatment can be described as a truly holistic treatment as it not only aids the release of physical tension but has been shown to work at an emotional level, calming the spirit, promoting relaxation, relieving the psychological of signs of anxiety and stress.

The benefits of IHM include:-

- Slowing down and deepening the breathing, which helps lower blood pressure.
- Promoting relaxation which can help with sleep.
- Improving the mood, helping to reduce stress and anxiety. It can also help with depression.
- Relieving muscular tension. This increases joint mobility, flexibility and improves posture.
- Relaxing and soothing aching muscles, helping to reduce stiffness.
- Increasing awareness of the mind-body connection to encourage feelings of wellbeing.
- Enhancing positive self-image.
- Promoting feelings of relaxation, focus, and happiness.

- Increasing alertness.
- Enhancing the capacity for calm thinking and creativity.
- Easing tension headaches, eye strain and ear problems.
- Helping with hair loss/thinning.

An IHM treatment at the Centre:-

- Takes 40-50 minutes.
- Is performed with the client seated in a normal low-backed chair.
- Is usually accompanied by relaxing music
- Aims to make the client feel comfortable and relaxed from the start.
- Is usually performed without oils, with client fully clothed. (Most clients prefer this).
- Can be performed with oils with appropriate clothes removed.
- Is generally a gentle treatment. (Most clients prefer this). Pressure can be increased if needed and agreed with the client.

Physical conditions IHM can treat:-

- Headaches
- Muscle and joint pains
- Muscle and joint mobility
- Eyestrain
- Sinus problems
- Insomnia
- Tinnitus
- Fatigue – physical

Emotional conditions IHM can treat:-

- Anxiety
- Stress and tension
- Fatigue – mental

Immediately following a treatment clients have reported:-

- Feeling calm and deeply relaxed from head to toe
- Reduction in tension in head, neck shoulders, chest
- An increase in joint mobility

At a follow-up treatment clients have reported:-

- Ongoing feeling of calm
- Increase in hair growth
- Decrease in hair loss
- Improved sleep
- Mental alertness; clearer thinking
- Less mental stress/tension
- Reduction in muscle pain/discomfort

The 'M' Technique

Developed and researched by Dr. Jane Buckle, the 'M' Technique evokes a rapid and profound relaxing effect. It consists of a series of stroking movements, performed in a set sequence and at a set pressure. The "M" Technique is particularly useful for persons who are fragile, or when massage is not appropriate, and has been enjoyed by clients who have experienced it at the Centre

Several therapists at the Centre now practise the technique and find it helpful for clients who want to experience therapeutic touch but are wary of massage or aromatherapy. The skills and content taught on the training course are suitable for health professionals, complementary therapists, and for anyone caring for someone with an advanced or chronic illness.

The "M" Technique is so light it can be used without any oil or lotion which is particularly helpful for people who are having radiotherapy. Other clients can experience this gentle therapy combined with their favourite aromatherapy blend. The "M" Technique can be carried out as a whole body treatment or on individual areas, for example, a face, neck and head session provides a lovely treatment.

Research published in 2008 showed that this technique had a different effect on the brain and was more relaxing than conventional massage. This effect has been evident in case- studies of clients with pre-operative anxiety, dermatological conditions and post-operative pain. Practitioners of disciplines such as the Bowen Technique, Reiki and Shiatsu have found the "M" Technique complements their existing therapies.

Case Study

This lady presented with ovarian cancer in 2007 and was already having chemotherapy. She had major surgery a few months later. Since that time she has had many chemotherapy treatments.

This lady has been having the 'M' Technique at the Centre for sometime now. She has said that the treatment helps her to feel at peace, calm and very relaxed. She has also said that the treatment improves her appetite, thus increasing her strength. At times she has been in considerable pain and on one occasion on a scale of one to ten, she was experiencing pain at 6 before the 'M' Technique treatment and at 3 afterwards.

The therapist says that she has found the 'M' Technique enjoyable to learn and a very effective treatment to use both on people in good health and on people with difficulties as in the case above.

Reference:

Jane Buckle Ph. D. R.N., Andrew Newberg M.D., Nancy Wintering M.S.W, Ellyn Hutton L.M., Catherine Lido Ph. D. and John Farrow, M.D., Ph.D.

Measurement of Regional Circular Blood Flow Associated with the 'M' Technique – Light Massage Therapy

Journal of Alternative and Complementary Medicine 2008 Volume 14

Physical Activities

The Walking Group

The walking Group was started in 2004 and was originally called the "Centre Strollers". The idea came about because it was thought beneficial for clients to get some exercise and fresh air to counteract the effects of some medical treatments. There was also the added benefit of being with people who would understand if some of the group couldn't walk as fast as others. The group met once a week except when the weather was too bad.

In the early days, the group met at different venues in Sutton Park but it was soon decided that it was less complicated if the meeting place was always the same and the Blackroot car park was the chosen venue. The meeting time was set at 10.00am every Wednesday and the walk was planned to finish by 11.30am approximately. The group always set off promptly at 10.05am, so attending promptly was encouraged, as standing around, especially in cold weather, and getting chilled could destroy the health benefits of the walk. In the case of heavy rain or snow, members telephone the group leader to check whether the walk is taking place.

The group would walk at the pace of the slowest walker and someone would always drop back if necessary to keep the slowest walker company. As time went on, it was found that people got better at walking, their pace increased and they were able to walk longer distances. The average distance used to be around 2.5 miles but, this increased, and now, sometimes 5 miles is achieved.

Being in Sutton Park in all seasons is very therapeutic because of the changing scenery and wildlife. Also, there is an absence of traffic noise and fumes.

Occasionally venues other than Sutton Park are chosen for special reasons, for example the bluebell woods at Middleton in May.

The group is quite large with a mixture of people, so that conversations are varied, informative and lively. There is no limit to numbers, so friends of Centre members have been able to join the group.

Sometimes a stop is made at the bistro after the walk and this adds to the feeling of wellbeing. A group lunch is arranged once a year.

What members say about the Walking Group:

"Fresh air, exercise and enjoyable company."

"Very good exercise with plenty of fresh air. We have great fun chatting. It is just what the doctor ordered, to keep me healthy and on top form."

"I look forward to the Wednesday walk. I like it because it is in the fresh air and you can connect with nature. Mixing with people with different views and knowledge enlightens me."

"I had never thought of the walk as being therapeutic. There is comfortable, informal companionship, laughter and understanding in a shared experience. There is easy chat which might include suggested remedies or discussion of ongoing or past treatments and experiences, but also talk of family and national events, almost anything. We mostly chat to whoever we are walking with, but this can vary in one morning. So, if there are 8 or 10 walkers that day, we will have an encounter with nearly everybody before we complete our walk an hour and a half later.

The leader chooses a different direction every week. We're now getting to know most of the acres quite well. We stick to paths and tracks, paths by the lakes and through the woods, over heath land and on a few occasions, in wet conditions, we stick to tarmac paths. Scarcely ever does the walk get cancelled due to bad weather conditions. Some prefer to walk quietly, observing the wild life and enjoying the changing seasons, the weather and the light. It is good to pause, savour the peace and quiet or watch the ponies. It is difficult to tell who is ill, who is between treatments or who is on the road to recovery, who is a carer, or who is bereaved. Walking is a great leveller. If someone needs to walk more slowly, the fitter and faster members will wait. The regular exercise has an effect on the way the group walks. We gradually get fitter and faster, better at hills and able to walk a little further each week and still get back on time. Yes, the Walking Group must be therapeutic, if you enjoy the outdoors. Spirits are lifted by the fresh air, companionship and exercise. Limbs, minds, hearts and lungs are exercised."

"Every Wednesday, a very dedicated group of people walk together. The leader encourages us forwards in all kinds of weather; we make sure we wear protective clothing and foot gear to withstand the wind and the rain. Since my husband was diagnosed with cancer, I have been attending the Cancer Support Centre. The benefit I am getting from the walking group is strength in body and mind. Strength makes life purposeful and productive. Regular exercise and walking promotes physical strength. Keeping the body strong and healthy, helps to keep the mind calm and serene. The Wednesday walk gives me both strength in the body and calmness in the mind. I would like to continue walking with the group as long as possible."

Yoga

Yoga is an ancient Indian practice for the improvement of body and mind. By practising Yoga, you can achieve a healthy body, calm attitude, mental strength and peace of mind. Because the practice of Yoga originated in the East, where hot temperatures discouraged vigorous exercise, the practice is more concerned with stretching.

The word yoga is derived from the Sanskrit word 'Yuj' which means to join or to yoke, therefore Yoga means union – union of the individual soul and reality.

The ancient yogis observed the movements of plants and animals and how they protected and defended themselves. They studied in particular the feline forms such as cats, lions and tigers and observed how they had very flexible spines. These movements were copied by the yogis and have been developed and refined over the years to make up the practice of hatha or physical yoga. Hatha is derived from 'Ha' which means the sun (the sun of your body is your soul) and 'Tha' which means moon and equates with consciousness. Yoga postures are called asanas and resemble living creatures, for example: the eagle or the cobra, and plants such as trees and flowers, for example the palm and the lotus flower. The postures positively exercise every part of the body.

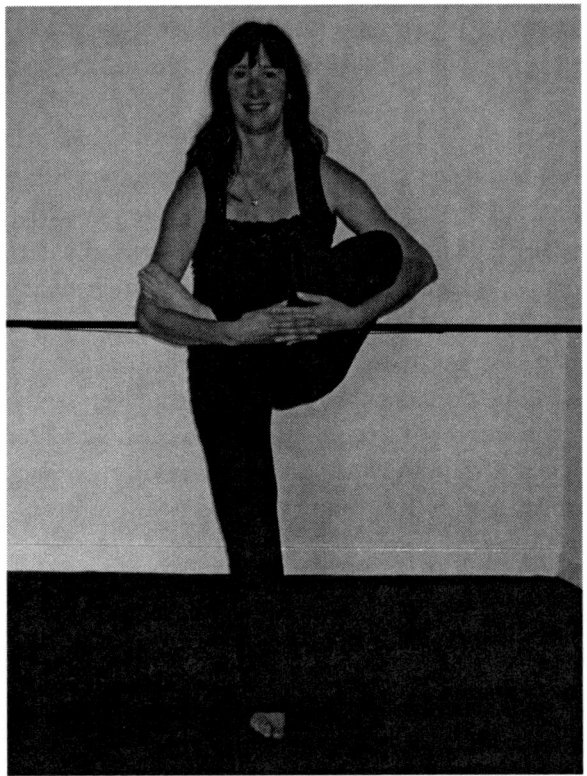

Yoga posture

The ancient yogi realised the importance of the spine which is the carrier of our vital nervous system and around which the body is built. The postures promote suppleness of the spine, a condition necessary for good health and for retaining youthfulness. The joints in the arms and legs are kept supple and all the muscles in the body are exercised and kept firm.

Yogis believe that deep and effective breathing is essential to health. The aim of yogic breathing is to calm and still the mind. Controlled yogic breathing exercises are called pranajamas. By breathing in a controlled manner, we can calm and eventually control our minds.

Yogis also practised a moral philosophy, the main tenets of which are:

- Moderation
- Kindness
- Positivity

These beliefs link with the philosophy of the Centre and the works Dr David Hamilton, Louise Hay, Bruce Lipton and others.

Hatha yoga classes have been offered at the Cancer Support Centre since 2009. Examples of postures practiced include 'full cat stretch' which straightens and stretches the spine, and the 'lion's roar' which is an excellent exercise for the throat and is believed to prevent colds. Some pranajamas (breathing exercises) are also practised. The lessons are adapted so that the less able clients can still participate; some of the exercises and postures are practised whilst sitting on a chair.

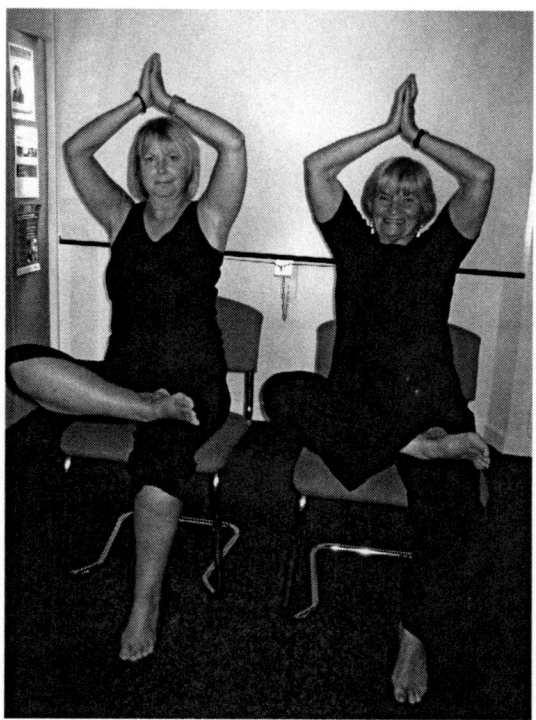

Yoga posture practised on a chair

A regular group of clients have found that yoga really works for them. They have practiced a range of postures and exercises and learned deep and effective breathing and how to switch off from thoughts and their daily routine. The benefits, they say, are increased suppleness and general wellbeing. The stretching exercises also help to release tension from the body and lead to a more relaxed and positive outlook on life. The postures also aid concentration and balance.

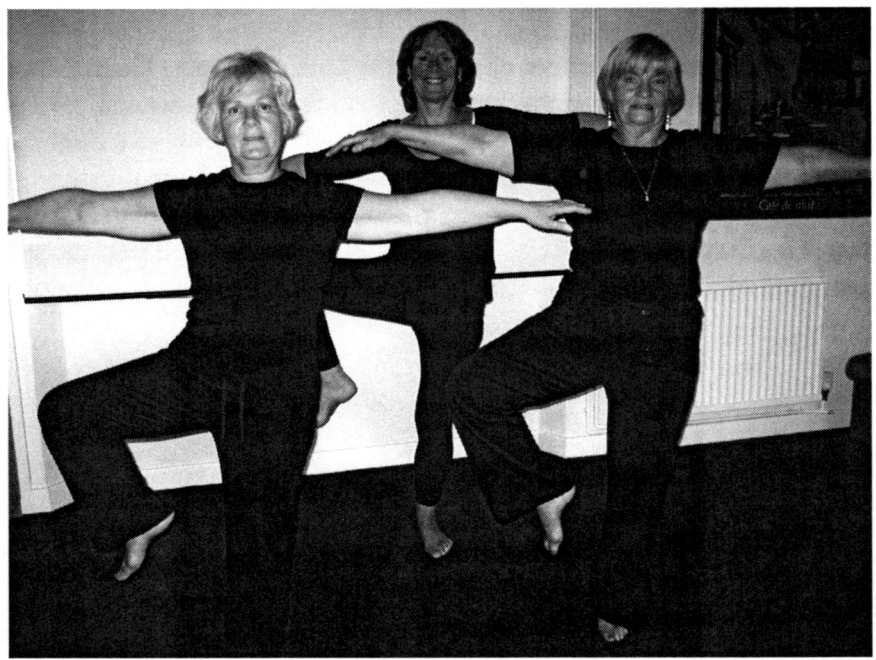

Yoga posture and balance

At the beginning of each lesson, there is a five minute period of relaxation when the group participants close their eyes and focus on their breathing. These five minute sessions are accompanied by relaxing music and positive and uplifting readings.

Every hatha yoga session has a theme such as 'animal poses' or 'yoga for complete health'. Yoga claims to have an exercise or posture for every single part of the body including the internal glands and organs.

At the end of each session the group is invited to lie down and put up their legs/feet to rest the heart. They adopt a 'partial upside down or inverted posture' which is considered by yogis to be essential to retain youthfulness. In this position a further five minute period of relaxation takes place.

The reactions of the ladies attending the group have been very positive:

"I feel strengthened, energised and yet relaxed with this class. A very special experience"

"I have recently joined the Yoga class and find it enjoyable and therapeutic. The leader is very welcoming and the session flows very well. I also feel I am benefitting from the exercises without it being too strenuous"

"I have been attending the Yoga group since my chemotherapy started. My body has changed a lot with the surgery and the after effects of the chemotherapy. Yoga allows me to stretch and move to a level I can manage. Through the months, I have got better at the postures and feel I can do so much more than I could. I try some of the postures at home too. I find the relaxation, meditation and poems that the teacher reads very helpful. The words give me strength to be positive and face the future with hope and enthusiasm. I am sure Yoga helps my internal organs as much as my muscles. I like the stretching as I feel it improves my posture and attitude to life. It is for everyone of all levels, so anyone can do it."

Creative Activities

The Art Group

Following the move to the larger premises at Station House, with the help of a generous grant from the Sharman Trust it was possible in 2004 to purchase the necessary materials and equipment to set up an art group. The Centre was fortunate to have a therapist, who had previously been an art teacher, who agreed to lead the group

Initially, in order to make the facility available to all clients, many of whom have a daytime job, the sessions were organised into eight week blocks which alternated between Monday mornings and Monday evenings. After a while it became clear that very few clients wished to make use of the evening sessions and those interested in joining the art group were able to attend the daytime group and so it has evolved into its present form. The group now meets regularly on Monday mornings. There would appear to be a core group of about eight to twelve clients at any one time, though the faces change as people leave for various reasons and new people join. Of course the numbers of clients present each week fluctuates. Indeed, as space is rather limited, it would be extremely difficult to accommodate the full group with a maximum of eight being preferable.

The aim has always been to provide a relaxed, welcoming atmosphere where clients of all abilities can feel secure enough to explore and develop their own creativity, at their own pace, but at the same time enjoy the company of others in a similar situation. Happily this appears to be the case and clients report that they find the whole experience very therapeutic. No pressure is placed on them to conform to any particular style, to use any particular material or to perform specific tasks; in fact quite the opposite is true. They are encouraged to follow their own interests and hopefully develop their own style, with guidance from the art teacher when needed.

A wide range of materials is available including: paints (acrylic, poster and watercolour), several types of pastels, crayons, inks, fabric paints/silk paints, wax/dyes for batik, printing inks/rollers etc. together with a well stocked resource area. All materials are provided free of charge to clients, although many are now so interested in the subject that they are collecting their own equipment and materials.

Clients are encouraged to retain all of their work even if they are not really happy with the outcome. This provides them with an excellent means of assessing their progress, something which is very satisfying for all concerned.

The following comments indicate how the clients value the group and the activities it provides:

"The best possible start to the week. Enjoyable and in good company. Our teacher is the best possible leader, always cheerful and supportive."

"I find coming to the art group relaxing as we do our own thing. Being on my own, the friendship here helps to take my mind off everyday problems."

"I hadn't picked up a paintbrush for 50 years and thought I couldn't draw or paint. At first, I was in shock from my diagnosis and treatment and could only fill pages with black paint and a red page of flames symbolising radiotherapy. Now, 17 months on, I can draw and paint bright, cheerful subjects such as animals, birds and seascapes. The teacher and the wonderful company of the art group do wonders to lift the spirits."

"I have found that this is one of the most relaxing pastimes I have taken up. The art class is 2 hours of friendship and total distraction from any problems. It is also possible to become so absorbed that I can actually pay no attention to the chatter. The teacher is the best possible, always willing to let you get on, on your own, whilst offering as much help as you need, always friendly, cheerful and totally supportive."

"Since loosing my husband to lung cancer after 45 years of marriage, I have found attending the art class each week very therapeutic. The group is very friendly and supportive and the teacher explains all the various techniques of art to me in simple form. I look forward to Monday. It is the highlight of my week."

"I find being a member of the group helps me to think of other things, and never having been very good at art, it is amusing to see some of the results. The group help me as we chat and joke about many things. Monday is a definite visit to the Centre for me, not to be missed if possible."

<u>Singing</u>

The value of music as a therapy has long been recognised and the Centre wished to offer this medium to the clients. As well as regular singing sessions, there have been talks and demonstrations from sound therapists and dancers and a ukulele player which were much appreciated by clients.

In recent years, two singing teachers have offered their services to the Centre. Each has offered a monthly singing lesson to a group of clients. These sessions were called 'Singing for Fun' on the programme as this was the aim: to provide an enjoyable experience whilst enabling relaxation and an improvement in breathing techniques.

Both teachers believed that anyone can learn to sing and part of each session involved learning to breathe correctly. The breathing techniques taught enhanced the singing but also had a lasting effect on good lung expansion. Filling the lungs completely is necessary for singing but is also beneficial for good health as filling the lungs with air rather than taking shallow breathes means that more oxygen is available to the body and this is essential for optimum cellular activity.

Both singing teachers taught singing to local choirs and some clients and volunteers enjoyed the singing so much that they joined one of the choirs so that they could sing more often.

The first teacher prepared his choir to perform concerts of various styles of music and offered to organise a concert to raise funds for the Centre. A number of the Centre's clients and volunteers took part in this and thoroughly enjoyed singing Verdi's 'Gloria'.

Both teachers arranged for their choirs to sing Christmas carols at large stores to raise funds for the Centre and again a number of clients and volunteers joined in. This was agreed to be a most enjoyable if rather cold experience.

One client wrote the following about singing at the Centre:

"I started going to the Cancer Support Centre while I was still receiving treatment for breast cancer. I noticed on the newsletter that there was a singing class, so I decided to go along. There was a good turnout and the atmosphere was great. It didn't matter if you could sing or not, it was a get together and cancer wasn't the reason you were there. It was all about feeling relaxed in yourself, throwing away your stress for a couple of hours with all the other women who knew what you were going through. I felt happy. It was great fun and I had a good dose of the feel good factor".

The Book Club

The book club, started in 2004, was the idea of one of the therapists and one of her clients, who found that their informal chats about the books they had read or were reading seemed to help relax the client when she was getting ready for her therapy, The chat continued after the therapy as well. The discussions often spilled over to the art group which the client attended; the therapist was also the art group leader. Other people in the art group also joined in and agreed that the art and the book chat was very relaxing and so the therapist and the client agreed to start the book club.

The book club met once a month and at the beginning, the suggestions about which books to read came from the members of the group. Each month a title was drawn from the suggestions made. The subjects suggested were extremely varied which led to lively debates. This method of selecting the books to read proved to create difficulties, as members could not always get the books from local libraries or afford to buy them and sometimes the suggestions for books to read dwindled. So, a new system was introduced whereby a quantity of books of the same title were borrowed from a local library and handed out at one meeting and returned at the next. One member, now the group leader, took responsibility for negotiating with the library, collecting and returning the books. Titles are suggested by members or by the librarians at Mere Green library, who have been most helpful and obliging. The club aims not to take advantage of the library by keeping books too long, but the library have been very understanding given members circumstances.

The group have read a wide selection of books, many of which, members admit, they would not have chosen to read. However, they have found them interesting and stimulating. Inevitably some authors that have been tried, few members would choose to read again.

At the monthly meeting, discussions about the current book take place and some of these have been quite lively and occasionally heated. The length of the meeting depends on how much interest has been raised by the book.

Membership of the Book Club has to be limited to 12, and there is a waiting list. The group has been largely made up of female clients with a few men involved. The group would value more male members. The lack of male members is a situation common to other activities at the Centre and to attendance generally.

Everyone involved over the years has said that they found reading for the Book Club, is a good way to take their minds off their anxieties and that it is stimulating; the meetings are invigorating, relaxing and often amusing.

<u>What Book Club members say</u>

"I have been introduced to many new authors, and I enjoy the discussion and support in congenial company."

"I have been encouraged to try a wide range of interesting books that I would not hitherto have considered. The subsequent discussion groups have been enjoyable, stimulating and have added an extra dimension to the reading experience".

"I am an avid reader of any types of book and thoroughly enjoy discussing the contents of the books. Also, it is very enjoyable to be with a group of people of the same mind."

Social Activities

From the early days of the Centre's existence, social activities have been seen as an important aspect for the wellbeing of both clients and volunteers and a variety of activities have been enjoyed. The aim of these activities was to provide an enjoyable experience which could be shared by clients and volunteers. They were an opportunity for people to get to know each other better and also a time to receive some support if needed. There was also an opportunity to forget worries and concerns for a time.

A house warming party was arranged when the Centre moved into Station House and another party for the Centre's fifth birthday. There has also been a dinner and dance to celebrate the tenth anniversary

Every Christmas a meal at a restaurant is arranged and these occasions have grown as the Centre has developed; so from groups of twenty or less, there may now be 60 to 80 attending these occasions.

There is also a Christmas party at the Centre every year, when lunch is shared and some in-house entertainment provided. Clients are encouraged to join in the entertainment if they wish. There is also the annual fundraising ball which some clients and volunteers choose to attend. Other fund raising events, such as quizzes, fairs and flower festivals also provide a social environment for all.

In 2004, 6 clients and 2 therapists spent a week in a French gite. This holiday benefitted everybody with visits to the beach every day, meals made and shared together and occasionally there was time for a little therapy.

A number of day and theatre trips have been arranged including a visit to the Houses of Parliament and a cruise on a canal boat. Film evenings have also been arranged at the Centre. Recently some of the meditation group members went on a trip to Glastonbury where they visited the Chalice Gardens and the Tor.

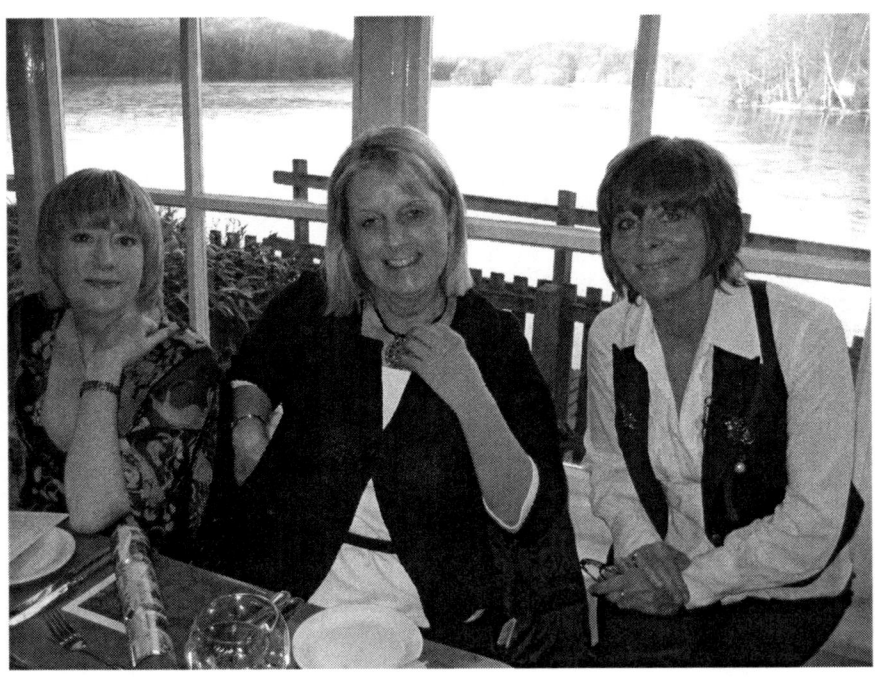

Christmas Lunch 2007

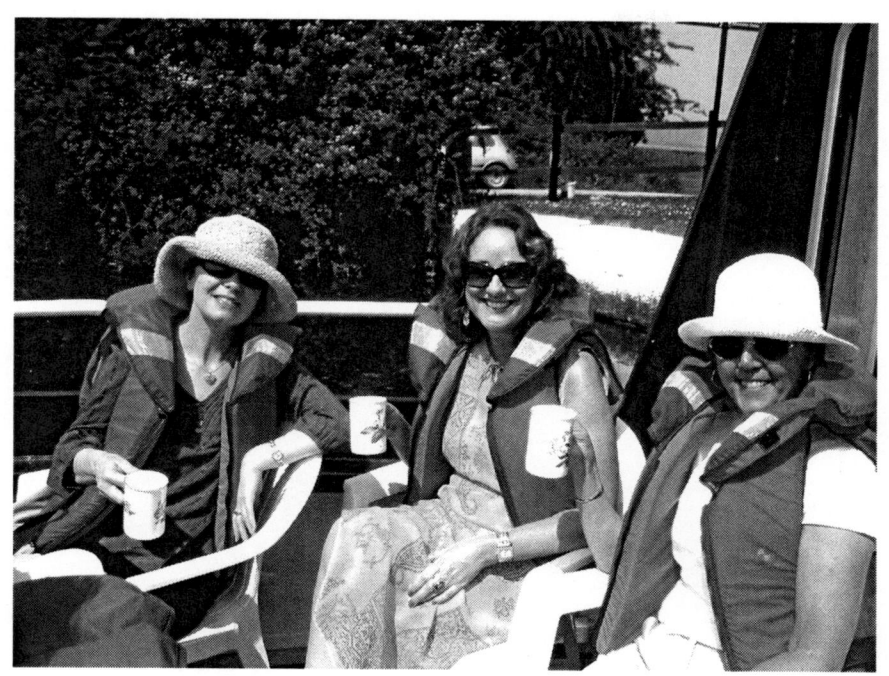

Canal Boat Trip

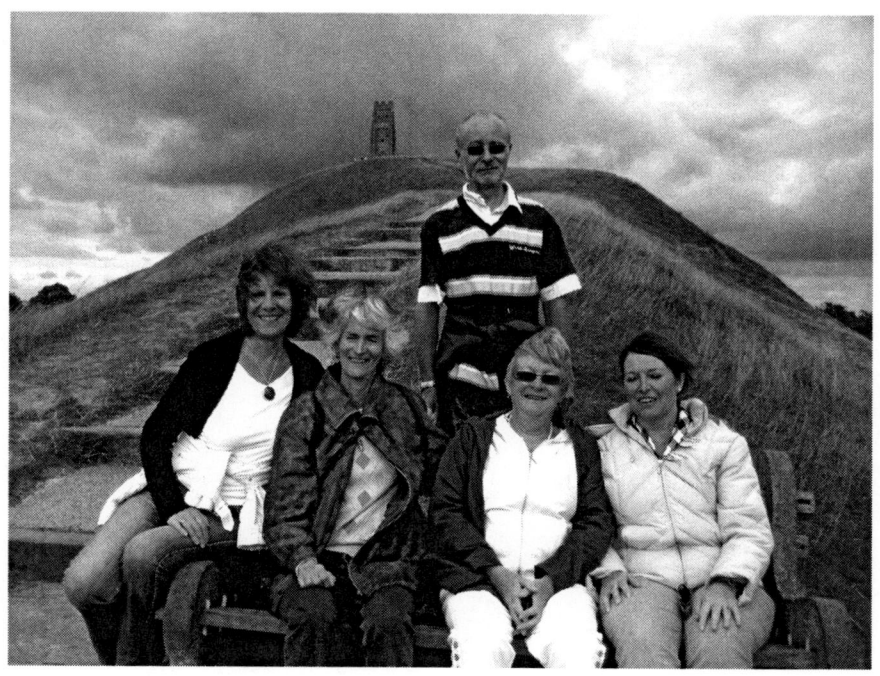

Meditation Group at Glastonbury Tor

Some of the regular group activities at the centre can also be seen as social events. Some clients find this aspect of the Centre's activities very helpful in their adjustment to their illness and perhaps a change of life style.

Ann's Story

Ann was diagnosed with ovarian cancer at the age of 23 and had surgery and chemotherapy. Obviously the diagnosis had a devastating effect on Ann and her family.

It was sometime after her diagnosis that Ann first came to the Cancer Support Centre. She had been finding it very hard to cope knowing that she would never be able to give birth to a child of her own. Ann participated in a number of the Centre's activities, joining various groups and attending Reiki courses. She made a number of friends who gave her great support. She also had counselling at the Centre.

Ann's family were also in need of the Centre's help, especially her mum and her sister. Her parents were divorced and her sister was a single mum with a young child. Both her mum and her sister were affected by Ann's diagnosis at such a young age, but they also had relationship and career difficulties.

The Centre offered help to Ann's mum and her sister with the result that the family were drawn closer together and they were able to come to terms with Ann's diagnosis and also get their lives together.

Ann desperately wanted to have a child, so she and her husband started to apply to be adoptive parents. This was a very challenging time for them both as the procedure is long and the outcome is never certain. The therapists at the Centre gave Ann as much support as they could during this time. Eventually Ann and Kevin were able to adopt a beautiful baby boy called Charlie. At the same time a friend from the Centre who was unable to have a child of her own also adopted a little boy and the friendship continued.

Charlie is now 5 years old and has started going to school.

Ann's Mum wrote to the local paper to express her gratitude to the Centre and this is what she said:

"Cancer does affect the whole family and I an sure if it wasn't for the genuine, constant support we received at the Centre, I would not be able to continue enjoying my family life today. I am so grateful for all their help at a time when our lives were at rock bottom."

The Role of Nutrition in Healing and Health

Introduction

Clients come to the Cancer Support Centre having some idea about the importance of good nutrition to their continuing health and wellbeing. They want to learn more at the Centre. Some of these clients have had hormone related cancers such as breast, ovarian or prostate, and are interested in following a dairy-free diet as recommended by Professor Jane Plant CBE. The Centre is fortunate to have Jane as a patron. When she visits, Jane is able to advise clients, therapists and volunteers about nutrition and also share the outcomes of her research.

The Centre recognises the importance of good nutrition for everyone's health and wellbeing, whether or not they have had cancer. The Centre and Jane would acknowledge that a nutritious diet helps with the prevention of many diseases and also aids recovery from disease and treatment.

Clients at the Centre are able to listen to informative talks about nutrition and use books from the library. The Centre is fortunate to have a naturopathic nutritional advisor to give individual advice to clients. However, it needs to be stressed that the Centre's philosophy is to empower clients by providing information and encouraging choice about dietary and lifestyle changes.

This chapter provides up-to-date information about healthy eating and drinking for those who wish to improve their diet including what to eat and what to avoid. For more individually tailored guidance, readers are advised to consult a qualified nutritional advisor.

Balanced diet:

Everyone needs a daily intake of fluids, carbohydrates, fats and proteins as well as vitamins, minerals, phytonutrients and dietary fibre. It is the amounts

85

and sources of these staple dietary constituents which will determine how healthy the diet is.

Natural unprocessed foods:

The diet should consist of foods in their natural state. A good diet should INCLUDE:

- whole grains
- fresh fruit, vegetables and herbs, preferably seasonal, organic and locally or home grown
- small amounts of organic or 'wild' animal protein
- seeds, nuts, beans, peas and lentils
- unrefined oils

and AVOID:

- processed foods, which contain refined ingredients and are nutrient poor

Carbohydrates

We need to eat carbohydrates to supply us with energy. Carbohydrates are broken down into simple sugars in the digestive tract. If we eat more than we need, fat will be deposited on the body. We obtain carbohydrates from grains, fruit and vegetables. Carbohydrates are produced by plants as a result of photosynthesis. Under the influence of sunlight, plants convert carbon dioxide and water into carbohydrate and oxygen.

Whole Grains:

Whole grains such as wholemeal flour and wholegrain rice are a healthy choice. Refined carbohydrates are best avoided as they have had their vitamins and minerals removed from them during processing. Examples of refined carbohydrates are white flour and white rice. White flour is found in many foods such as white bread, cakes, biscuits, pizzas and pies.

Glutinous Grains:

Some people benefit from removing glutinous grains from their diet. Glutinous grains are wheat, rye, oats and barley. A trial period without these grains, or perhaps initially just wheat, may result in less digestive problems and improved wellbeing. Less glutinous grains are whole grain rice, millet and quinoa. Another alternative is buckwheat which is a seed not a grain. Short grain brown rice, cooked slowly and chewed well, is easily digested. It is a neutral, hydrating and non challenging food.

Fruit and vegetables and sugar:

Fruit and vegetables are excellent sources of carbohydrates. Five portions every day is the minimum that should be eaten but aiming for ten portions a day will enhance health and wellbeing. Green vegetables such as broccoli, cabbage, kale, spinach and watercress should be eaten every day.

Fruit contains sugar and some vegetables, such as carrots, sweet potato and butternut squash, also have a high sugar content. A healthy diet should contain sugar from these foods and not white sugar which has no nutritional value.

White sugar is found in many foods such as jam, breakfast cereals, cakes, biscuits and chocolate bars. When white sugar is eaten, it is quickly broken down in the digestive system and then absorbed into the blood. The pancreas produces higher amounts of insulin to remove the sugar from the blood. When it has been removed, blood sugar levels drop dramatically. This can produce symptoms such as low energy, dizziness, an inability to concentrate, headaches and nausea. Avoiding sugary foods and eating small regular meals containing proteins and oils and complex carbohydrates such as whole grains will help to keep blood sugar stable. Drinking water at regular intervals will also prove helpful.

Alternatives to white sugar are those sugars which contain nutrients such as raw cane sugar and maple syrup or sugars contained in fruit and vegetables such as butternut squash. Consider baking your own cakes and look for recipes containing these alternatives. Avoid substituting white sugar with commercially made non-sugar sweeteners such as aspartame, which contain chemicals that can be harmful to health.

Clients with active cancer should look upon home-made cakes and desserts as 'treats' and limit them to two modest servings per week.

Vitamins and Minerals

The body is unable to make either vitamins or minerals and they must be obtained in the diet from plants. Some vitamins and minerals can be obtained from meat and fish.

There are around 22 essential minerals and many are involved in body metabolism, nervous system functioning, bone health and water balance. The richest sources will be found in plants grown in high quality soils rich in micro-organisms that convert the minerals into a form that the plants can take up.

Vitamins are vital for life as they are necessary for growth and development, body metabolism and physical well being. B vitamins and vitamin C are water soluble and cannot be stored in the body. Fat soluble vitamins are Vitamins A, D, E and K. They are carried around the body in oils and fats and any excess is stored in the liver and fatty tissues.

Vitamins will be more plentiful in fruit which is picked and eaten when ripe and with the least time spent in transit and storage. Similarly, vegetables are best eaten as fresh as possible. Vegetables should be lightly cooked to preserve nutrients. Steaming is the best method and the water can be used for stocks and sauces.

Certain minerals such as selenium and zinc, and vitamins such as Vitamin E, Vitamin C and beta-carotene are helpful in the prevention of cancer and the treatment of some types of cancer. This is due to their anti-oxidant properties (see explanation below).

Phytonutrients

The term 'phytonutrient' literally means 'plant-based' nutrient. Another word used is 'phytochemical'. These are compounds in plant foods which are not considered essential, like vitamins and minerals. They have health-promoting and health-enhancing benefits such as being anti-oxidant, anti-inflammatory, anti-viral and anti-fungal. They form part of plants' immune systems, protecting them against conditions such as disease, injury and harsh weather. Scientists are discovering and identifying new phytochemicals and a small number are used to make chemo-therapy drugs to combat cancer. Herbal preparations also contain phytonutrients.

Different classifications of phytonutrients are isoflavones, flavenoids or bioflavenoids, phytosterols, carotenoids, indoles, organic sulphur compounds and curciminoids. Many are claimed by scientists to have anti-cancer properties. Four examples are:

- Isoflavones are found in soya and foods made from soy. They are also found in small amount in clover sprouts, chickpeas, some types of beans, split peas, lentils and green tea. Isoflavones are weak oestrogens that bind to oestrogen receptors of the body's cells and prevent harmful oestrogens from attaching to the receptors. Clients with oestrogen related cancers should include these foods in their diet.
- Catechins are flavenoids found in green tea. They have been found to be effective against UV induced skin cancer.
- Indole-3-carbinol is an indole found in cabbage, Brussels sprouts, kale and broccoli. It has many anti-cancer benefits including stopping cancer cells growing and increasing the death rate of cancer cells.
- Allicin is an organic sulphur compound found in garlic. Allicin restricts the blood supply to cancer tumours and stops them growing.

Anti-oxidants

Anti-oxidants neutralise free radicals which cause healthy cells to weaken and eventually lead to disease. Brightly coloured fruits and vegetables contain anti-oxidants. Some examples are:

- Yellow and orange colours: found in carrots, butternut squash, pumpkin and sweet potato. These foods are high in beta-carotene from which the body makes Vitamin A. Vitamin A is associated with good eyesight, healthy cell membranes and immune function.
- Red, blue and purple colours: found in blueberries, raspberries, strawberries, red cabbage, beetroot and grape skin. These colours are the result of anthocyanins which provide protection to DNA, reduce

the growth rate of cancer cells, are anti-inflammatory, increase white cell numbers and inhibit cancer enzymes.

- Red colour: found in tomatoes, pink grapefruit, apricots, red oranges, watermelon and rosehips. These foods contain lycopene which is thought to lower the risk of prostrate cancer.

Eating a plentiful and broad range of plant foods containing many phytonutrients, which work together beneficially in the body, is the key to good health. There is now considerable evidence that diets rich in whole grains, fruit, vegetables, herbs and spices help people to maintain the lowest risk of disease.

Fibre

Fibre is obtained from whole grains, pulses such as lentils, vegetables and fruit. It is necessary for the digestive system to process and absorb nutrients in food. Fibre is required to enable food to travel through the digestive tract in a timely way and to produce soft, bulky stools. A plant-based diet helps to maintain the balance of good bacteria to bad bacteria in the digestive tract. As a large amount of the immune system operates in the digestive system, fibre is necessary to good health.

Proteins

There are 20 different amino acids found in proteins. Eight of these are essential amino acids as they must be obtained from food and cannot be made or stored in the body. Protein helps build and repair body tissues and assists in making enzymes, hormones, and other body chemicals which are vital for optimal health. Proteins are the necessary building blocks of bones, muscles, cartilage, skin, hair, nails and blood.

Animal protein contains the full range of amino acids needed in an adult's diet. Beef, pork and foods made from these meats such as ham, sausages, mincemeat and beef-burgers should be avoided. Lamb is a better choice but again should be eaten sparingly. These red meats are acid forming and take longer to digest and make their way through the body than other meats. Chicken is a better choice of animal protein. Choose organic meats and meat from wild animals which will provide a more natural diet. Health experts now tell us eggs are a good choice of animal protein and can be eaten regularly. Again, choose organic.

Fish is a good source of animal protein. Oily fish such as wild salmon, mackerel, herring, tuna, trout and sardines should be eaten once or twice per week and white fish once per week. Shellfish is also a good source of protein and low in fat.

Protein is also obtained from non-animal foods such as beans (e.g. red kidney, haricot, butter, pinto and soy), and peas e.g. 'garden' peas, split peas, chickpeas and lentils. These should be eaten with a grain to provide a full range of essential amino acids e.g. whole grain rice or wholemeal toast. Grains contain some protein, as well as containing carbohydrate. Soy products such as tofu and tempeh are also good sources of protein. Traditionally beans and peas would have comprised up to 30% of the British diet but nowadays the average diet contains around 3%. More of these 'legumes' in the diet and less animal protein will create a more balanced diet.

Seeds, such as sesame, sunflower, pumpkin and flax, and nuts, such as almonds, walnuts, hazelnuts and Brazil nuts, are also sources of amino acids that make up proteins. These can be eaten at breakfast, as snacks during the day, sprinkled on salads or as an ingredient of main meals. Nuts and seeds are more easily digested if they are crushed or ground up and have been soaked for several hours.

Large amounts of protein are not required in the diet although protein at every meal helps to keep blood sugar stable. Health professionals suggest men should eat 55.5g (grams) of protein per day and women 45g. The daily diet should contain 25% of food obtained from protein.

Professor Jane Plant CBE, the Centre's patron, recommends, for the prevention of cancer, that the daily diet should contain no more than 10% of animal meat which should be thoroughly cooked. Animal meat contains natural hormones and growth factors and may also contain carcinogenic man-made chemicals including harmful oestrogens; Jane also recommends avoiding farmed fish, especially salmon, and fish liver oils.

Jane Plant's advice to people with active cancers is that animal protein in the diet should be completely avoided.

Oils and Fats

Unsaturated fats

These oils, which are liquid at room temperature, should form the majority of oils in the diet. They are obtained from oily fish and the seeds of plants and contain various amounts of Omega 3, Omega 6 and Omega 9.

Omega 3 and Omega 6 are referred to as essential fatty acids (EFAs) as they cannot be made by the body and have to be obtained from the diet.

EFAs have many functions in the body. They:

*   support the cardiovascular, reproductive, immune, and nervous systems.
*   manufacture and repair cell membranes so the cells can properly absorb nutrients and expel harmful waste products.
*   produce prostaglandins (short-lived tissue hormones), which regulate body functions such as heart rate, blood pressure, blood clotting, fertility, conception, and play a role in immune function by regulating inflammation and encouraging the body to fight infection.

EFAs have to be obtained in the correct amounts and also in the correct ratio of Omega 3 to Omega 6 which is between 1:1 and 1:4. Modern diets contain very high amounts of Omega 6 and low amounts of Omega 3. EFA deficiency and Omega 6/3 imbalance is linked with depression and serious health conditions including cancer.

A diet supplying the correct balance and amounts of Omega 6 and Omega 3 will include:

*   Omega 3 from oily fish e.g. salmon, mackerel, sardines and also halibut and shrimp
*   Omega 3 from flaxseeds (linseeds) ground up or chewed well or one tablespoon of organic flax oil per day. Flax seed oil can contain up to 58% Omega 3.

- Omega 3 in smaller amounts can be obtained from hemp seed oil (20%), rape seed oil (7%), soybean oil (7%), walnut oil (5%) and wheat germ oil (5%), pumpkin oil (0-15%) and rice bran oil (1%).
- Supplementing the diet with Omega 3 capsules from the flesh of fish (not the liver where toxins are concentrated) is advisable.
- Small amounts of omega 3 can be found in kale, spinach and avocado.
- Omega 6 is found in many seed oils such as hemp oil (60%), sunflower oil (65%), sesame seed oil (45%), and evening primrose oil (81%).

Processed foods should be avoided as they contain large amounts of Omega 6. Meats from animals which are fed grains contain large amounts of Omega 6. Eating meat from grass fed animals is a better choice.

Omega 9 is not an EFA as the body is able to make small amounts. Omega 9 is found in many seed oils but the main source is olive oil. The health benefits of the Mediterranean diet, which includes olive oil, are well known. Olive oil reduces the risk of heart disease and Spanish researchers have found it reduces the risk of colon cancer.

Saturated fats

These fats are solid at room temperature. Saturated fats from animals especially beef, pork and lamb should be avoided or minimised. Saturated fats from plants such as coconut oil, palm oil and cocoa are beneficial to health and can be eaten in small amounts. A small amount of butter, which is easily digested, may be included in the diet.

Unrefined oils and refined oils

Choose oils which are produced using traditional methods and are labelled in the following ways: cold pressed, extra virgin, virgin, unrefined or organic. All other oils will have been subjected to processing methods such as degumming, refining, bleaching and deodorizing which remove nutrients such as fatty acids, vitamins and minerals.

Hydrogenation and transfats

Avoid oils which have been hydrogenated. This process makes oils solid such as found in margarines and shortenings found in processed foods.

Not only will these fats have had nutrients removed but their molecules will have been altered. Avoid transfats, which are damaging to the cells of the body. Fortunately, many manufacturers are removing these from their foods as the implications for poor health have been recognised. However, transfats may still be used in the catering trade.

Containers and storage

Buy unrefined oils in glass bottles. Chemicals can leach from plastic into oils. Choose tinted glass as oils can degrade when exposed to light. Store bottled oils in a cool, dark place and do not exceed the sell by date. Once opened, consume oils as soon as possible. Always replace the tops of bottles securely to avoid oxygen degrading oils. Rancid oils are damaging to health.

Cooking with oils

Avoid cooking with unrefined, unsaturated oils containing Omega 3, Omega 6 and Omega 9. Virgin and extra virgin olive oils are damaged above a temperature of 140 degrees Celsius. Add unrefined oils, including olive oil, to raw foods or when foods have been cooked.

Use extra virgin coconut oil, organic butter, ghee, duck or goose fat for cooking. These saturated fats are not damaged when heated. Fats should never be so hot that they smoke. Coconut oil is excellent for use in stir fries. Onions can be softened by heating olive with water to keep the temperature around 100C. Potatoes can be roasted in goose or duck fat. Vegetables can be roasted in coconut oil or butter.

Dairy products and oestrogen related cancer

Dairy products, plentiful in a typical 'British' diet, contain fat as well as protein. However, there is considerable scientific evidence on the role of dairy produce in promoting disease – not only breast, prostate, ovarian and other cancers but also other health problems from allergic reactions to osteoporosis and diabetes. Professor Jane Plant's book, 'Your Life in Your Hands' explains the dangers of eating dairy produce for people with oestrogen related cancers and also promotes a dairy free diet for prevention of these types of cancer. The Vegetarian and Vegan Foundation has published two reports 'White Lies - the consequences of consuming cow's milk' and also 'One in Nine' which provide additional information.

The above recommend that dairy produce including butter, margarine, milk, cream and cheese should be omitted from the diet by clients with oestrogen related cancers as they may contain hormones which promote cancer growth. Goat's milk and goat's cheese are also in this category. Duck and goose fat is also best avoided as are foods that contain dairy products such as cakes, puddings and biscuits.

Alternatives to cow's milk are organic soya milk, rice milk and almond milk. For cooking, extra virgin coconut oil is the best alternative. Olive oil can replace butter on bread. There are also various nut butters for sale in supermarkets or health food shops.

Readers who do not wish to omit dairy produce totally from their diet should consider avoiding milk and cheese. Small amounts of organic, unsalted butter and organic natural live yoghurt are better choices.

N.B. Soy can inhibit the uptake of iodine which is needed for a healthy-functioning thyroid and for every cell in the body. If eating soya products, make sure that iodine rich foods, such as in seaweeds, are included in the diet, or supplement with kelp capsules. Those who are prescribed thyroxin should seek advice from their G.P. or specialist.

Calories in fats and oils

The total intake of all fat and oil should comprise no more than 20% of the total daily diet.

One gram of fat = 9 calories, whereas one gram of protein and one gram of carbohydrates = 4 calories each.

If a 100g product is 300 calories of energy in total and its fat content is 10g, it may be advertised as 10% fat. But using calories as a measure, 10g of fat = 90 calories. This is nearly 30% of the total energy content – not 10%.

Beware of hidden fats!

<u>Alkalising Diet:</u>

The body must have an internal alkaline environment. The blood has to operate within a very narrow range which is slightly alkaline otherwise death will result. Body tissues also operate within an alkaline environment but if they become slightly acid, they will not function optimally and symptoms of disease will manifest. Long term acidity of the tissues can lead to various degenerative diseases, one being cancer.

The body can become acidic due to various factors such as emotional and physical stress and exposure to toxins and radiation. Another major factor is a poor diet. Exposure to these stresses should be minimised.

To change body tissues from acid to alkaline, the diet should comprise 80% alkaline and 20% acid forming foods. For a 'maintenance' diet the diet should be 70% alkaline and 30% acid. These percentages relate to the amount of acid and alkaline foods on your plate. The most acid forming foods are red meats and shellfish, glutinous grains (wheat, rye, oats and barley), dairy foods, and processed foods such as cakes and pastries. The most alkaline foods are vegetables, fruit and soy milk. Seeds, obtainable from health food stores, and sprouted in water at home are very nutritious and very alkalising. Freshly made juices from vegetables and some fruit are also very alkalising. Vegetables soups also help to alkalise the body tissues.

Note: A well-functioning digestive system converts citrus fruits, such as blueberries, cranberries and prunes, from acid to alkaline. People with poor digestion may have difficulty converting these types of fruit and may become more acidic. Until their digestion improves, these people may be advised to include only the juice of lemons and limes.

Suggested daily menu for a healthy diet:

Breakfast:

- Fresh juice e.g. apples, carrots, celery, celeriac, fennel, cucumber, small portion of beetroot, a few hearts of Romaine lettuce leaves.

and

- Nuts and seeds, ground and soaked, plus a wholegrain and raisins with soya, rice or almond milk. (Alternative to wheat, rye, oats or barley whole grains are flakes of rice, buckwheat, millet or quinoa, which are obtainable from some supermarkets and health food shops.)

or

- Poached egg with short grain brown rice and steamed spinach

Lunch:

- Salad (of a variety of colours e.g. hearts of Romaine lettuce, watercress, rocket, fennel, celery, cucumber, radish, red pepper, tomato, red onion, beetroot) with avocado, walnuts and apple served with quinoa. Add extra virgin olive oil and apple cider vinegar.

or

- Salad (of a variety of colours) with sardines served with rice. Add extra virgin olive oil and apple cider vinegar.

or

- Salad (of a variety of colours) with marinated cubes of tofu fried in extra virgin coconut oil and rice noodles.

or

- Home-made soup. Suggestions: Use lentils or beans or a little fish or organic chicken; spices such as cumin, coriander and fresh ginger;

fresh vegetables such as onions, garlic, leeks, root vegetables (e.g carrots, celeriac, parsnip, turnip, greens). Add to the finished soup chopped fresh herbs such as parsley, coriander, basil or chives.

Dinner:

- Stir fry using organic chicken or tofu and fresh vegetables (e.g peppers, courgettes, carrots, celery, spring onions) with rice noodles fried in extra virgin coconut oil.

or

- Grilled fish with fresh greens (i.e. cabbage, broccoli, Brussels sprouts and kale), carrots, courgettes, leeks and baked sweet potato.

or

- Lentil chilli with added vegetables, red kidney beans and served with whole grain rice.

Suppers:

- Blinis or pancakes made with buckwheat flour and spread with hummus or tahini. (Both available from good supermarkets and health food shops.)

Or

- protein drink (available from health food shops) made with water

Or

- Smoothie made with natural organic yoghurt or soya yoghurt, one teaspoon of bee pollen and one teaspoon of flax oil.

These can also be eaten at breakfast time.

<u>Snacks:</u>

+ Nuts, seeds, fresh fruit, raisins

+ Vegetables (e.g. carrots, cucumber, celery) with dips such as humous, tahini or tzatziki (made with natural organic yoghurt or soya yoghurt, cucumber and mint).

<u>Fluids</u>

<u>Water</u>

Although considered last in this chapter this is absolutely vital to life and needs to be consumed in appropriate amounts.

Water is essential to life and the amount and quality of the water we drink can determine how healthy we are and our avoidance of disease. The human body is composed of 60% to 85% water and water is present in every body fluid i.e. blood, lymph, digestive juices, mucous and joint fluids. Water is also inside every cell and between the cells. It is needed to transport oxygen, nutrients including vitamins and minerals and also hormones and enzymes into the cells. It is also vital for the removal of waste products and toxins from the cells and from the body.

The body uses approximately 5 pints/3 litres of water a day to excrete toxins and waste via the kidneys, bowel, skin (perspiration) and lungs (water vapour). Therefore the daily intake of water must be at least 5 pints to replace the water excreted from the body. When toxins have accumulated due to insufficient intake, higher amounts of water daily are required. When fluid intake includes other substances such as caffeine, tannin, sugars, alcohol, additives and colourings, the water in which they are dissolved will not count as pure water as it will be required to transport and excrete the solutes already in it. Pure water needs to be consumed in addition to these other fluids, ideally 5 to 6 pints daily.

The build up of waste products and toxins in and around the cells inhibits the movement of oxygen and nutrients into the cells and can lead to many types of disease.

Sources of water:

Tap water is derived from various sources in nature, collected into reservoirs, filtered to remove large particles and treated with chlorine to remove dangerous micro-organisms. In some areas, fluoride is added to the water supply with the aim of preventing dental decay. However, fluoride is known to be toxic to humans and can also cause dental problems, so many people would prefer not to have it in their water supply. Treatment of tap water does not remove unwanted chemicals such as pesticides and waste from chemical processes, heavy metals and oestrogens derived from water courses. Chlorine is toxic to the body. Pipes in old buildings can contain lead which can pollute the water supply.

Bottled water is available from various springs (mineral water) both from the British Isles and abroad. The substances dissolved in these waters will vary depending on the water source and the process of preparation for bottling. Some bottled waters are produced by reprocessing municipal water. Most plastic bottles will leach chemicals, which may be carcinogenic, into the water gradually and especially after opening or being kept in a warm place. Glass bottles are preferable. Filtration of tap water can improve quality of water by removing some or most of the harmful substances from the water. Jug filters are one method but these need to be emptied and cleaned regularly to prevent multiplication of micro-organisms. Filters must be changed as recommended. Glass filter jugs are preferable to plastic for the same reasons as above. Boiling the water after filtration is another choice.

Reverse Osmosis Filtration is an effective and cost effective way of filtration of domestic water. A good system can remove 90+% of harmful chemicals, heavy metals, chlorine, fluoride and micro-organisms. Useful minerals may also be removed but in the latest systems these can be returned to the water. It is important that the system is well maintained and filters changed as advised. Systems are made of hard plastics which are less likely to leach chemicals.

Other Fluids

Drinks to include in a healthy diet are: green tea, ginger tea made with fresh lemon and fresh ginger, fruit teas, home-made juice and almond milk and rice milk.

Drink sparingly black leaf tea, Earl Grey and soya milk.

Drinks to avoid are: coffee, alcohol, long-life cartons of orange and fruit juices, water flavoured with artificial sweeteners, all drinks made with cow's milk, drinks containing high amounts of sugar, carbonated 'fizzy' drinks.

<u>Tips for Healthy Eating and Drinking</u>

- Eat at least 8 portions of fruit & vegetables a day including greens such as cabbage, broccoli, spinach and watercress.
- Try making juices and smoothies with fresh fruit & vegetables to achieve 10 portions a day.
- Use organic and locally sourced food if possible.
- Lightly steam vegetables and other foods to maintain vitamin content
- Drink at least 2 litres of water daily in addition to other caffeine – free and sugar – free drinks to hydrate cells and remove toxins.
- Drink filtered water if possible. Try a jug filter to begin with – a glass one preferably. Ideally fit a Reverse osmosis filter to your kitchen sink.
- Avoid black tea & coffee as they contain caffeine. Try other teas including green, white (which is believed to have anti-cancer properties), Rooibos (Red Bush Tea), fruit and herbal teas.
- Reduce or cut out alcohol, especially wines which contain sodium sulphite.
- Avoid red meat. Small amounts of organic chicken and fish are acceptable as are organic, free range eggs. A little organic, hill raised lamb can be consumed occasionally.
- Include pulses, i.e. peas, beans and lentils, cooked or sprouted, in your diet as these are a source of protein.
- Remove dairy foods and milk from the diet, especially if suffering from breast, ovarian, testicular or prostate cancer
- Remove animal fats, hydrogenated oils, trans-fats and cooking oils in plastic bottles from your diet.
- Use organic coconut oil for cooking at high temperatures. Add water to heated olive oil to soften onions for soups, stews and casseroles.
- Add extra virgin olive oil to cooked foods. Do not use for cooking as it is easily damaged.
- Eat oily fish, a good source of Omega 3, once or twice per week.

- Include nuts and seeds in the diet as they are a good source of protein and omega oils
- Supplement the daily diet with good quality omega 3 capsules and/ or cold pressed flax oil. (Do not supplement if taking the drug, Warfarin).
- Use whole grains and cereals including short grain brown rice, quinoa and millet, avoiding wheat.
- Avoid salt, white and refined sugar and artificial sweeteners such as aspartame in food.
- Avoid all processed and pre-packaged meals.
- Read the small print.

References

Professor Jane Plant	2007 Your Life in Your Hands, Virgin
	2005 The Plant Programme Virgin
	2010 Eating For Better Health, Virgin
Dr Justine Butler	2006 White Lies
	2007 One in Nine
	The Vegetarian and Vegan Foundation

Acupuncture

What is Acupuncture?

Acupuncture is an ancient Chinese medicine founded on the philosophy that within each of us exists the flow of a life energy called Qi (pronounced chee). It has been developed, improved and enhanced over several 1000 years and is a common medical practice in eastern countries, comfortably used in conjunction with Western medicine.

The philosophy explains that within our body runs a network of energy channels (meridians) along which Qi flows internally and externally. This flow aids the body's healthy function and maintains a glorious balance between the mind, body and soul. It is when this flow stops or becomes hindered that illness results and can be affected by a number of factors. These include physical and emotional trauma, stress, diet, lifestyle and environmental factors for example living in a damp, cold house. Illness can then manifest either as an external condition, for instance affecting the skin, muscles or joints, or an internal disharmony - anxiety, insomnia, stomach issues etc.

Along the meridian lines (energy channels) are specific markers called acupuncture points. These are junctions which are needled to stimulate the energy to flow again and thus regain the balance of the body. Of interest mummies have been found in eastern mountains with basic acupuncture points tattooed on there preserved bodies. This suggests that the ancient Chinese shared their knowledge when travelling from village to village and literally marked the points on themselves in order to preserve the wisdom.

There are literally 100s of points on the body. These exist on a network of channels which flow internally and externally, which means that a positive affect can be achieved by needling away from the problem area. To clarify, if a person has a stomach problem then one point to assist with stomach function is located on the legs!

This makes acupuncture an accessible treatment for people with all sorts of health issues. Within cancer care, where there may have been surgery or removal of lymph glands, this is a particularly practical and versatile therapy to achieve results.

How acupuncture is used in Cancer Care.

Acupuncture is about rebalancing the body and restoring health. Specific complaints that are treatable at the Cancer Support Centre are as follows

In no particular order these are:

- Nausea - Heartburn
- Flushes and Night Sweats
- Pain
- Sinus Relief
- Anxiety and Stress
- Post-operative Scarring - tightening of the tissue can create tension with surrounding tissue which then may cause pain and discomfort. This can be softened and relaxed.
- Fatigue and Anaemia
- Muscle pain, Tension and Heavy Limbs
- Headaches and Muzzy Heads
- Insomnia: This is sometimes difficult to shift; it depends what the cause is.

Of course the level of response to the treatment varies on an individual basis depending on so many different factors, such as: medication, treatment, diet, lifestyle, family support.

Contraindications - When Acupuncture Can Not be Used

- Lymphedema - This is the big needle no, no! Whichever limb the lymph nodes have been removed from then NO needling is allowed along that arm, finger, leg etc. However, there is a school of thought in Chinese acupuncture that by needling the opposite limb it will stimulate an affect on the other side any way. I have seen evidence of this in clinic when a client has stated they have felt a sensation in the exact same needle location but on the opposite side of there body!

- Surgery - Naturally if there are any scars still healing then treatment within this area is avoided.

- Skin rashes - If the skin is broken, hot, swollen then direct needling into the area is contraindicated. However, it is possible to needle around the affected area, just not in it.

Some Case Studies from the Cancer Support Centre

1. A young lady in her mid 30s had had surgery and a lot of chemotherapy for a rare cancer in her abdomen. She made wonderful progress but after treatment suffered horrendous hot flushes and night sweats. She was encouraged to receive hormone treatment, but decided to delay the option for a few months and decided to have acupuncture. After a time not only did her hot flushes and sweats clear but her periods returned. A couple of years later she now has a lovely son much to the amazement of the medical profession.

2. During her chemotherapy cycle, a lady came for treatment for hot flushes. However, it turned out she was also suffering from chemotherapy triggered sinus and headache (muzziness) problems. This was duly treated and after one session her sinuses had cleared and her head muzziness improved.

3. A teenage girl was receiving medical treatment and was suffering from terrible nausea. She did not wish to have acupuncture but after a short chat it was decided she could wear some travel sickness pressure bands. These press on a specific acupuncture points and gently stimulate the point without need for needling. She was shown exactly where to put them and how to find the acupuncture pressure point. A few days later her mother phoned to say that her sickness had significantly reduced.

Reference

Angela Hicks   2007   The Acupuncture Handbook:
How Acupuncture Works and
How It Can Help You
Piatkus Books Ltd

Faith's Story

Faith first came to the centre in 2005, following surgery for an abdominal tumour, which was finally confirmed to be Ewings sarcoma, a rare and aggressive form of cancer.

Faith had symptoms of indigestion and reflux for 3 years prior to the surgery, but despite having endoscopies and other tests, no diagnosis was made until shortly before the surgery when a scan showed the tumour. An operation was planned but before this could happen, Faith collapsed and was rushed to hospital in a critical condition having lost a lot of blood. Blood transfusion was attempted but at first the transfusion of blood was difficult and Faith's life was in the balance. Thankfully following the use of a blood warmer, the transfusion was successful and Faith survived. However, the planned operation was now more essential and was undertaken by two expert surgeons, a gastroenterologist and a gynaecologist, because the tumour was surrounding organs in both regions. During the surgery, a portion of intestine was removed but fortunately Faith did not need the colostomy she had been warned about. One ovary and its Fallopian tube were found to be twisted and damaged but they were not removed. Specimens of the tumour were sent to laboratories in England but the tumour could not be categorically identified so a specimen was sent to the USA and finally the diagnosis of Ewings sarcoma was made.

Faith was referred to a specialist in this type of tumour and she was told that she would have to have intensive chemotherapy. Although Faith was a young woman and the chemotherapy would inevitably make her sterile, she was told that there was no time to harvest her eggs for later use. So, the chemotherapy commenced. Faith spent 5 days in hospital every third week having a combination of 4 different chemotherapy drugs, each giving very unpleasant side effects, meaning that there was only one week in three that Faith felt relatively normal.. Faith was told that she should have 15 cycles of the chemotherapy but that very few people stayed the course; however

Faith did. It was during this time that Faith came to the Cancer Support Centre. During the weeks when she was not having chemotherapy she attended the Centre for complementary therapies; she received counselling, Reiki and hypnotherapy. Soon the effects of the chemotherapy on Faiths body resulted in frequent hot flushes and bad night sweats and it was at this time that acupuncture was commenced which had a very good effect on the sweats and flushes. She also suffered with acne at this time, and this also responded to the acupuncture.

Because of the intensive chemotherapy, Faith's doctors assumed that she was in the menopause and suggested that she should commence hormone replacement therapy (HRT). Faith was not happy about this and she saw two different fertility doctors both of whom did tests to confirm that she was in the menopause. Again HRT was suggested but Faith, after consulting her General Practitioner (GP), decided not to take any more medication for another six months.

During this time Faith had returned to work but found it hard to cope emotionally and so the Centre offered more counselling which proved to be very helpful.

As Faith began to feel better, she met a new partner and fell in love. As the relationship progressed, Faith told her partner that she would not be able to have children. He was very disappointed about this as he wanted to have children, but he loved Faith and stayed with her.

Early in 2009, Faith began to feel unwell. She had queasiness, nausea and vomiting, which she put down to the large amount of Gogi berries (a healthy fruit) she had been eating. However the symptoms persisted and she feared a reoccurrence of the cancer. Eventually Faith consulted her GP who suggested that, before any other tests, she should do a pregnancy test. This, much to Faith and her partner's surprise and shock, proved to be positive and a normal pregnancy and natural water birth followed. In November 2009, a beautiful and healthy baby boy arrived to the great delight of Faith and her partner.

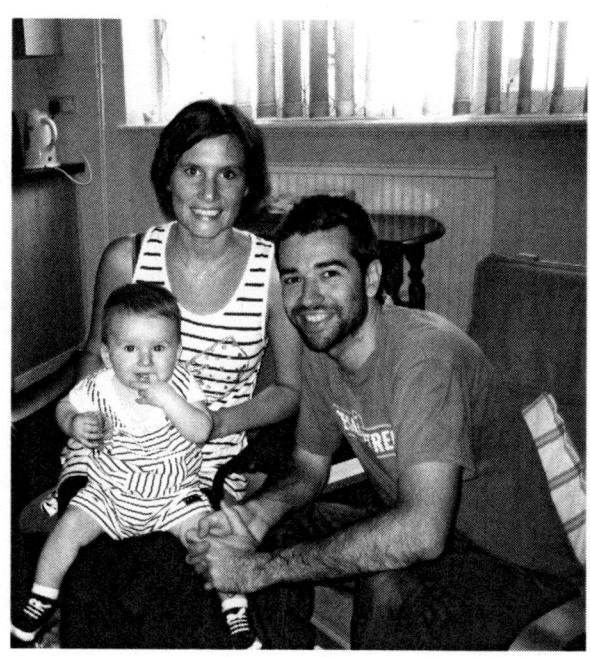

Faith, Kingsley and Fion

Faith says that the help and support the Centre gave to her was "massive". It made her feel she was not alone and relieved both physical and psychological symptoms. Faith's mum, who was devastated by Faith's illness, also received counselling and support at the Centre. She is now a very proud grandmother.

Homoeopathy

Homoeopathy is a holistic method of treatment for symptoms and diseases. The remedies chosen are based on a wide consideration of how the individual is as a person. The homoeopath will carefully collect information from the client, not only about the symptoms of the disease but also about previous experiences and behaviours, emotional and psychological state, and environmental, social and genetic factors. The personality type of the client will also be considered.

The principles of homoeopathy were discovered by a German doctor, Samuel Hahnemann in the late 18th century. Working as a translator, to fund his study of chemistry, one of his tasks was to translate a major medical textbook at the time, known as Cullen's Materia Medica. Whilst doing this he found out that although many remedies used at that time were ineffective, some did actually work. One of these was the bark of the Cinchona tree, which was used to treat 'swamp fever', now known as malaria. This bark substance, used for malaria, is now known as Quinine. Hahnemann wondered how the bark could work and experimented on himself, discovering that he developed symptoms of a fever. He had stumbled on the 'law of similars' which is the main principle of homeopathy today and means that 'like cures like'. He realised that the substance which causes symptoms in a healthy person can cure those same symptoms in illness. An example of this is: insomnia may be treated with a remedy called coffea which is made from coffee.

Hahnemann then went on to investigate the ability of other substances to induce symptoms. He found that many of the substances were toxic and so he turned his mind to how they might be diluted. He discovered that the diluted substances retained the ability to cause symptoms so they could be used safely to treat illness. In fact he found that by further diluting the substances and vibrating the solution each time, the diluted substance seemed to gain power.

Today, homoeopathic remedies are prepared by serial dilution with shaking by forceful striking, which homoeopaths call 'succussion', after each dilution. The most diluted homoeopathic remedies are believed to be the most potent in relieving symptoms. The effect of dilution and succession is termed 'potentization. Some people find it hard to believe that, this dilution of a substance until it is untraceable in the solution, can be effective. Hahnemann, however believed that succussion activated the vital energy of the solution. Homoeopaths believe that the remedies trigger the immune system into action.

In 2000, the House of Lords Select Committee on Science and Technology cited homoeopathy as one of the five Group1 therapies having "an individual diagnostic approach". The other four were osteopathy, chiropractic, herbal medicine and acupuncture.

Hahnemann eventually produced his own materia medica, called Materia Medica Pura, but his work has been expanded on considerably over the last 200 years and there are now over 2000 recognised homoeopathic remedies. Homeopaths still use materia medicas and they have also over the years developed repertories. Repertories list symptoms according to parts or systems of the body and include lists of all the remedies known to have an effect on each symptom. The popularity of homoeopathy as a method of treatment is now expanding rapidly and a significant number of medical doctors also practice homoeopathy, so it can be seen as a complementary medicine.

One way in which homoeopathy differs from general medicine is in the length of consultation. The homoeopath will spend an hour or more collecting all the information needed to determine which remedy is appropriate for the individual, whereas general practitioners' consultations are usually limited to about six minutes. Clients often find this longer consultation time reassuring as they are able to talk fully about their symptoms and problems.

Homoeopathy is one of the few complementary therapies where, a substance is prescribed for ingestion, but given the manner in which the remedies are prepared the chances of side effects are minimal. Homoeopathic remedies will not affect the effect of medicines prescribed by the doctor but the prescribed medicines may limit the effect of the remedies.

Clients at the Cancer Support Centre have found homoeopathy beneficial for a number of symptoms and conditions related to their illness and medical and surgical treatment. Homoeopathy, as other therapies at the Centre, is seen as complementary to medical treatment, but clients can continue to benefit from homoeopathy when medical treatment has been completed. Remedies prescribed before surgery can assist in reducing inflammation, bruising and pain and accelerate healing.

Homoeopathy has been used at the Cancer Centre, to treat clients with the following symptoms:

- Sleeplessness
- Lack of energy and chronic tiredness
- Headaches
- Anxiety and fears
- Night sweats and hot flushes caused by, either an early menopause due to surgery or treatment, or treatment for prostate cancer
- Digestive disorders
- Recurring respiratory disorders
- Wound healing
- Allergies

References

Dr Andrew Lockie   1999   The Family Guide to Homoeopathy
                               Hamish Hamilton Ltd.
The House of Lords Select Committee on Science and Technology (1999-2000) 6th Report): The Stationary Office 2000

Bowen Technique

The Bowen Technique was pioneered by a man called Tom Bowen (1916–1982). Tom grew up in Geelong, Australia where his parents had moved a few years before his birth. He came from a working-class background and he started his first job as a manual labourer. While he was developing his therapy in Australia in the 1950s and 1960s, he was fascinated by the different postures people had and how this related to their symptoms of ill-health or muscle pain, etc.

Tom had an uncanny ability to observe how people walked, sat and moved. He drew remarkable accurate conclusions as to the root cause of their pain. His fascination with bodywork was born out of a desire to help people who were suffering. Tom Bowen did not promote or teach his technique and he only allowed a very small number of therapists to observe him working. However he did work closely with some associates, most notably his secretary, Irene Horwood and osteopaths Ossie and Elaine Rentsch, who he entrusted to document his work.

The Bowen Technique is a non-invasive holistic therapy consisting of a sequence of gentle moves over muscles and soft connective tissue, interspersed with short periods of rest to allow the body to respond. The treatment takes approximately 45 minutes to an hour and most work can be applied through light clothing. The Bowen Technique is not a massage and is generally considered to be a safe and effective tool, particularly useful when other treatments are unsuitable. This is especially the case in acute or severe conditions where the client is very elderly or infirm and it can help to improve the quality of life, for the terminally ill.

The Bowen Technique encourages re-alignment of the body, whilst promoting a deep sense of relaxation, helping people to lead a more comfortable and fulfilling life.

The Bowen Technique has a good record in treating:

* Anxiety and stress related conditions.
* Back pain, sciatic and spinal problems.
* Digestive and bowel problems such as Irritable Bowel Syndrome.
* Headaches and migraine.
* Asthma and respiratory conditions.
* Whiplash injuries.
* Joint problems such as tennis elbow, frozen shoulder, ankle and knee injuries.
* Infant colic, bedwetting.
* Repetitive Strain Injury and Carpal Tunnel Syndrome.
* Sports injuries.
* Hay fever and ear and sinus problems.
* Chronic fatigue.
* Lymphatic drainage.

The benefit of the Bowen Technique for people with cancer is a relaxing and lasting experience from a treatment that uses a gentle, hands-on, holistic approach, helping to reduce feelings of anxiety and stress as well as pain, at a vulnerable time. Clients with cancer may suffer from any of the ailments listed above as a result of the cancer and its treatment or as a separate condition which will exacerbate the effects of the cancer if not relieved. Sometimes carers of those with cancer may suffer from the any of the above ailments and this may affect their caring role so the Centre may offer therapies to carers in this situation.

The Bowen Technique as an established and recognised therapy, has gone from strength to strength since it introduction into the UK in the early 1990's and has now be accepted for The Complementary and Natural Healthcare Council (CNHC) registration from Monday, 15th February, 2010.

Examples of how Bowen Technique has helped clients

Client 1

This lady originally came for treatment, presenting with lower back pain, following numerous surgeries. She found, from the first night after treatment, she was sleeping better, which has remained the case and she also reported feeling more positive in her self. The lower back pain eased and resolved itself over the coming days.

The client resumed treatment 6 months later after the lower back pain came back suddenly whilst bending over to pick something up. She has since had regular treatment after under going a single Mastectomy in August 2009 followed by another Mastectomy a month later. The regular follow up treatments now are as much to address the lymphatic drainage as muscular skeletal problems.

The client says:

"My first encounter with Bowen was quite a while ago now and I remember that as the session progressed I thought 'how can something so gentle and relaxing have an effect on the mechanics of my body?' Well, I soon found out, after sleeping like a baby that night I awoke next morning with a positive lightness and spring in my step.

Since then, over a period time, I have had Bowen treatment many times. I had thought that with age came the aches and pains and we just had to put up with them. Not so, a Bowen treatment or two certainly makes a huge difference to my general well being as well as specific muscular problems.

Unfortunately in 2009 I was diagnosed with a re-occurrence of the cancer and two mastectomies were performed. Having declined the medical route for treatment, I chose to go the holistic way in which Bowen plays a big ongoing part; the treatments to help with mobility and lymphatic drainage. I now think of Bowen as a regular part of my treatment and it gives me a tremendous feeling of security".

Client 2

This gentleman came for treatment, presenting with severely restricted movement in the Pelvic area, following radiation treatment through the side of the hips to treat prostrate cancer. This resulted in him being unable to walk or stand normally, or get in and out of chairs unaided.

The client says:

"From the very first treatment I felt an overwhelming sense of confidence that things were going to be okay and my mobility started to improve straight away and has continued to improve following each treatment.

The Bowen treatment has made me more confident and pushed the cancer to the back of my mind and I'm now even managing to walk without the aid of a stick. I am also able to dress myself (although I still need some help to put my socks on) and going up and down stairs un-aided is a vast move forward from where I was."

I'm sure, with the ongoing treatment, my mobility will continue to improve, even to the point that I can put my own socks on. Thank you to the Bowen practitioner for all the help and understanding and to the Cancer Support Centre, for all their wonderful support".

Client 3

This lady came for treatment, presenting with a frozen right shoulder, experiencing severely restricted movement in all directions. She also had lower back pain, which was resolved after six treatments. She has since had two top up treatments and the shoulder and lower back work improvement has been maintained.

The clients says:

"Having muscles that had been weakened by months of inactivity before and following bowel cancer, inadvertently led to my old back problem reoccurring. The frozen shoulder, with total restriction, caused by simply reaching for something in the back of the car, just created further mobility problems.

Finding Bowen turned out to be a revelation and I have no doubt the Bowen treatment shortened the muscle recovery time (which I had been told could be up to 2 years) massively. Sleeping is now better and I find I can lie in any position without any discomfort, a vast improvement on previously

Muscle strength has now virtually returned allowing swimming and gardening activities to be resumed. In fact it is hard now to remember ever having a frozen shoulder, never mind a bad back".

Reference

Julian Baker   2002 The Bowen Technique,
                            Corpus Publishing

Education and Training for Clients, Volunteers and Therapists

Education and Training has always featured in the Cancer Centre's activities. The philosophy states that access to information is empowering and the Centre also promotes continuous education for staff, volunteers and therapists. Although sometimes therapists and volunteers are encouraged to attend training events outside of the Centre, many training activities have taken place in house.

Volunteers and therapists have attended 'Introduction to Counselling Skills' courses at the Centre, where the emphasis has been on the listening and responding to those affected by cancer. The Centre is fortunate to have several counsellors with training qualifications working at the Centre. These courses are very much valued by those who attended them.

Many of the clients, volunteers and therapists have attended Reiki 1 and Reiki 2 courses and a few have become Reiki masters.

The Heal Your Life courses have been run regularly, primarily for clients but some volunteers and therapists have attended the courses for their own personal development.

In addition to the above courses, there have been regular talks and short courses aimed at informing clients about the choices they might make to change to a healthy lifestyle, including eating and drinking to promote health and avoid cancer. These talks and courses have been delivered by the Centre's therapists and nutritional advisor and also by outside experts in these topics.

In the early days of the Centre's development, therapists, all of whom had qualifications in their own particular therapy/therapies, were encouraged and supported to attend professional courses to increase their knowledge about offering their therapies to those affected by cancer. Following attendance of such a course, the therapist was requested to give feedback to other therapists who might benefit from the new information gleaned.

During the ten years since the Centre opened, the therapists have organised regular sessions at the Centre, where the sharing of information would enable the updating of knowledge and techniques related to of their own therapies as well as those of their colleagues. These training sessions were of benefit to all therapists and enabled them to refer clients for appropriate therapies and promote the holistic approach to healing.

As the Centre developed, increasing the variety of therapies used and recognising how much the holistic approach was benefitting the clients, it was decided that the skills and expertise at the Centre needed to be shared with other therapists working with clients affected by cancer. So, in recent years, weekend courses have been offered and targeted at therapists from other organisations. These have covered the range of therapies used at the Centre, their application and examples of case studies of clients who have benefitted from the various therapies. These courses have been very much valued by those who attended them.

Some years ago the Centre purchased videos and books so that therapists at the Centre could attend video workshops to learn Quantum Touch. The majority of the therapists attended these workshops and two therapists went onto become certified therapists. This enabled them to conduct video workshops for therapists from other centres and to arrange further taught courses at the Centre to enable others to progress to gain certification.

One therapist gained support to attend 'M' Technique training and also a course to become an 'M' Technique teacher. This therapist now provides training courses for therapists at the Centre and also for those from other organisations

The trustees and therapists at the Centre strongly support the educational ethic and believe that the Centre could extend its educational courses to teach the community at large to live healthily and avoid cancer and other serious illness.

Tips for Healthy Living and for Recovery from Disease & Treatment

There is a massive amount of information on this subject. Here are some of the changes you might like to make in your daily life in order to enhance your health and wellbeing

Relaxation

Relaxation is vital in our lives and aids healing. You may already have your own ways of relaxing, but you can learn meditation, relaxation and creative visualisation techniques in many places. Alternatively follow the scripts in Chapter 4.

Sleep

It is important to get adequate sleep as it is during sleep that most healing takes place. Sleeping well in the early part of the night is also important. If you have difficulty getting to sleep, try the following:

- Have your main meal earlier in the day and eat just a small amount of carbohydrate such as porridge before retiring. If you wake up regularly during the night, reducing or leaving out the carbohydrate and eating a small amount of protein before retiring may be helpful
- Have a relaxing bath before going to bed
- Use lavender oil in your bath or on your pillow
- Listen to some relaxing music or a relaxation tape/CD
- Sleep in complete darkness
- Remove as many electrical devices as possible from your bedroom
- Remove your clock from your bedroom so that you cannot keep checking the time

Exercise

It is well recognised that exercise is good for us mentally and physically. Find forms of exercise which appeal to you and are within your capabilities. Walking, swimming and dancing are good. Joining a gym, health club or playing a particular sport are all good but may not appeal to everybody. You could join a yoga class for good all-round exercise.

Complementary therapies

Complementary therapies can benefit you in many ways, from aiding relaxation and giving you the feel good factor to dealing with the effects of treatment and enhancing healing and well being.

Bath Products and Cosmetics

Many of these contain toxic substances which could be absorbed through the skin. These include aluminium, SLES (Sodium Lauryl Sulphate) and parabens as well as propellants. Crystal deodorants are an alternative to spray deodorants which contain propellants and roll on deodorants which may contain aluminium. You might like to switch to a healthy, non-fluoride toothpaste as fluoride is a toxic substance.

Household Cleaning products

Again, many of these contain toxins and propellants which can pollute the atmosphere and be inhaled or absorbed by those in the house. A number of companies now produce healthier products.

Environmental Pollution

It is impossible to avoid this totally but try to avoid smoky and chemically polluted environments. Use mobile phones and wire free equipment as little as possible. Switch off electrical appliances when not in use. You can use crystals to absorb electro-magnetic energy and there are radiation protection covers for mobile phones. Avoid carpets and furnishings protected by chemicals. Stop using microwave ovens for cooking.

Final Thoughts

Throughout this book, holistic healing of mind body and spirit has been the theme. Reflecting on the book, I recognise that there is another dimension which has hardly been mentioned.

Those of us who conceived the idea of a cancer support centre were driven by a desire to help and support those affected by cancer. To this end we gave of our time and resources and developed what we have today. Therapists who joined the Centre worked conscientiously for the benefit of the clients and gave much more in time and effort than was expected of them. Volunteers also had the same ethic. On reflection, I would suggest that what they all gave was love. One therapy in particular, Reiki, has been described as giving love and I am sure that the way in which the all therapists and volunteers have supported their clients was with love. "Heal Your Life" (Louise Hay) workshops at the Centre emphasise the value of loving yourself and other talks and workshops have echoed this theme. When you love yourself then you have the capacity to love others.

The original aim of the founders of the Centre was to provide a place of sanctuary and support for those affected by cancer and this has been fulfilled by the relaxing and caring atmosphere which has developed in the Centre. I would suggest that many clients feel loved and cared for at the Centre.

When clients meet together in groups to participate in one of the Centre's activities, they make friends and a genuine sense of caring develops between members of the group; it could be said that they share love with each other.

David Hamilton, in "Why kindness is Good for You" (2010) demonstrates how kindness is good for the giver and the receiver. I would suggest that most acts of kindness are fuelled by is love. In "It's The Thought that Counts",

David, suggests that in love is" the power to change the world", we should express "love for self", "love for others" and "love for nature".

Reference

Dr David Hamilton   2006 It's the Thought That Counts,
Hay House

2010 Why Kindness is Good for You,
Hay House

Love Meditation

- Find a quiet, relaxing place where you will not be disturbed
- Focus on your breathing, deepening and slowing breathing to a relaxed rhythm
- As you breathe in focus on breathing in love
- As you breathe out focus letting go of hurt, hate, bitterness, anger
- As you breathe in feel love circulating to every cell of your body. May be you can see the cells light up as they absorb love
- Focus on breathing in love for yourself
- Feel the glow of light and warmth of love in your body and cells
- When you feel full of love for yourself you can breathe out love for all those close to you
- Continue to breathe in love
- Breathe out love for those in your wider circle of friends and those in your community
- See and sense that love going out to all
- Send love to those you do not know who are in great need of love
- Reflect again on the warmth and light of the love within you
- Send out love to all parts of our world and the universe beyond
- Feel again that warmth and depth of love for yourself
- Reactivate these feelings of love regularly

About the Editor

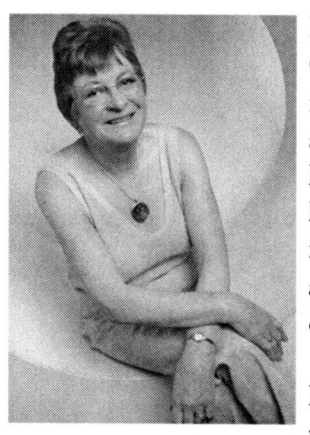

Mavis Cunningham MA, BEd. founded the Cancer Support Centre-Sutton Coldfield in 2000. Prior to training as a therapist, she practiced, first as a nurse and later as a lecturer in nursing. She has been a counsellor, hypnotherapist and supervisor of therapists for almost 20 years. She supports therapists at the Cancer Support Centre and organises developmental training courses for them.

Mavis is passionate about helping people to heal physically, emotionally and psychologically. She believes that if people adopted the ways of living suggested in the book, many cases of cancer and other serious illnesses could be prevented.

Lightning Source UK Ltd.
Milton Keynes UK
27 January 2011

166503UK00001B/16/P